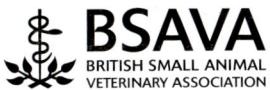

BSAVA
BRITISH SMALL ANIMAL
VETERINARY ASSOCIATION

BSAVA Guide to
Procedures
in Small Animal Practice
2nd edition

Editors:

Nick Bexfield BVetMed PhD DSAM DipECVIM-CA CBiol FSB MRCVS
European Specialist in Small Animal Internal Medicine

Clinical Associate Professor in Small Animal Medicine and Oncology
School of Veterinary Medicine and Science
University of Nottingham, Sutton Bonington Campus, Leicestershire LE12 5RD

and

Karla Lee MA VetMB PhD CertSAS DipECVS PGCAP FHEA MRCVS
European Specialist in Small Animal Surgery

Senior Lecturer in Small Animal Surgery
Clinical Science and Services
The Royal Veterinary College, University of London, Hawkshead Lane,
Hatfield, Hertfordshire AL9 7TA

Published by:

British Small Animal Veterinary Association
Woodrow House, 1 Telford Way,
Waterwells Business Park, Quedgeley,
Gloucester GL2 2AB

A Company Limited by Guarantee in England
Registered Company No. 2837793
Registered as a Charity

First edition 2010
Reprinted with corrections 2011
Second edition 2014
Copyright © 2014 BSAVA

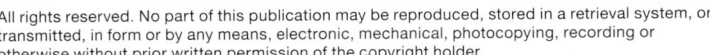

D1807208

The illustrations in this Guide were drawn by S.J. Elmhurst BA Hons (www.livingart.org.uk) and are printed with her permission.

A catalogue record for this book is available from the British Library.

ISBN 978 1 905319 67 1

The publishers, editors and contributors cannot take responsibility for information provided on dosages and methods of application of drugs mentioned or referred to in this publication. Details of this kind must be verified in each case by individual users from up to date literature published by the manufacturers or suppliers of those drugs. Veterinary surgeons are reminded that in each case they must follow all appropriate national legislation and regulations (for example, in the United Kingdom, the prescribing cascade) from time to time in force.

Printed in India by Imprint Digital
Printed on ECF paper made from sustainable forests

2456MDC14

Other titles from BSAVA

Manual of Canine & Feline Abdominal Imaging
Manual of Canine & Feline Abdominal Surgery
Manual of Canine & Feline Advanced Veterinary Nursing
Manual of Canine & Feline Anaesthesia and Analgesia
Manual of Canine & Feline Behavioural Medicine
Manual of Canine & Feline Cardiorespiratory Medicine
Manual of Canine & Feline Clinical Pathology
Manual of Canine & Feline Dentistry
Manual of Canine & Feline Dermatology
Manual of Canine & Feline Emergency and Critical Care
Manual of Canine & Feline Endocrinology
Manual of Canine & Feline Endoscopy and Endosurgery
Manual of Canine & Feline Gastroenterology
Manual of Canine & Feline Haematology and Transfusion Medicine
Manual of Canine & Feline Head, Neck and Thoracic Surgery
Manual of Canine & Feline Infectious Diseases
Manual of Canine & Feline Musculoskeletal Disorders
Manual of Canine & Feline Musculoskeletal Imaging
Manual of Canine & Feline Nephrology and Urology
Manual of Canine & Feline Neurology
Manual of Canine & Feline Oncology
Manual of Canine & Feline Ophthalmology
Manual of Canine & Feline Radiography and Radiology:
    A Foundation Manual
Manual of Canine & Feline Rehabilitation, Supportive and Palliative Care:
    Case Studies in Patient Management
Manual of Canine & Feline Reproduction and Neonatology
Manual of Canine & Feline Surgical Principles: A Foundation Manual
Manual of Canine & Feline Thoracic Imaging
Manual of Canine & Feline Wound Management and Reconstruction
Manual of Canine & Feline Ultrasonography
Manual of Exotic Pet and Wildlife Nursing
Manual of Exotic Pets: A Foundation Manual
Manual of Feline Practice: A Foundation Manual
Manual of Ornamental Fish
Manual of Practical Animal Care
Manual of Practical Veterinary Nursing
Manual of Psittacine Birds
Manual of Rabbit Medicine
Manual of Rabbit Surgery, Dentistry and Imaging
Manual of Raptors, Pigeons and Passerine Birds
Manual of Reptiles
Manual of Rodents and Ferrets
Manual of Small Animal Fracture Repair and Management
Manual of Small Animal Practice Management and Development
Manual of Wildlife Casualties
Pocketbook for Veterinary Nurses
Pocketbook for Vets

Small Animal Formulary
Every member of BSAVA receives a complimentary copy of the Formulary as part of their membership benefits or has access to an online edition

For further information on these and all BSAVA publications, please visit our website: www.bsava.com

Contents

System examinations

Procedures A to Z

Foreword

The first edition of the *BSAVA Guide to Procedures in Small Animal Practice* (2010) has proven to be one of the most popular BSAVA membership benefits and has become a key practice reference source in hard copy, pdf or app format.

Editors Nick Bexfield and Karla Lee have worked tirelessly to produce this updated second edition of the 'procedures guide'. This new edition continues to offer practitioners very practical, step-by-step guidance on how to perform the most important diagnostic and therapeutic procedures in small animal practice.

The second edition has a new, eye-catching and user-friendly design, including the use of full colour photographs. New techniques featured include how to perform the edrophonium response test, gall bladder aspiration, gastric decontamination and peritoneal dialysis. The important guides to body system examinations have been relocated to the front of the book, and the second edition is now fully indexed.

No matter whether you use the guide as a spiral-bound hard copy, or as an app on your mobile device, I am sure that you will continue to find this book an invaluable resource in day-to-day practice.

Professor Michael J. Day
BSc BVMS(Hons) PhD DSc DipECVP FASM FRCPath FRCVS

BSAVA President 2013–2014

Preface

It is our pleasure to introduce to you the second edition of the *BSAVA Guide to Procedures in Small Animal Practice*, which has been written for veterinary surgeons, veterinary nurses and students. We have been delighted by the success of the first edition, which suggests that this Guide has become the number one reference for step-by-step instructions on diagnostic and therapeutic procedures performed routinely in small animal veterinary practice. The second edition aims to build on this success, to increase the confidence and accuracy with which these procedures are performed, by responding directly to the feedback we have received from the BSAVA readership.

We have reviewed and updated all the procedures in the Guide in line with new editions of BSAVA Manuals and with progress in the field of veterinary medicine. We have consolidated the clinical examination protocols for body systems into a separate dedicated section. New procedures for this edition include the Edrophonium response test, Gall bladder aspiration, Gastric decontamination, Local anaesthesia and Peritoneal dialysis. Many procedures now benefit from the addition of colour diagrams and photographs, to clarify and really bring to life the procedures we describe. And the addition of an Index will make it easier to find just what you are looking for.

We are once again indebted to the innumerable contributors who have written procedures within the BSAVA Manuals on which we have drawn. We are also grateful to our colleagues who have reviewed procedures within this edition, including Dan Chan, Charlotte Dawson, Ed Ives, Elvin Kulendra, Sorrel Langley-Hobbs, Nic Rousset, Joel Silva, An Vanhaesebrouck, Holger Volk and Penny Watson. We are especially grateful to Jaime Viscasillas for his contribution to the Local anaesthesia procedure, which we hope will increase the practice of these important analgesic techniques in clinical practice. We would also like to thank Samantha Elmhurst for her illustrations, and our numerous colleagues who have contributed images or assisted in acquiring them specifically for this Guide. Finally, we would like to thank the Publishing team at BSAVA for their patience and attention to detail, without which this Guide would not have been possible.

Nick Bexfield
Karla Lee

January 2014

Cardiorespiratory examination

Indications/Use

- Successful management of the animal with cardiorespiratory disease depends on accurate anatomical localization of disease and efficient diagnostic planning
- Determination of the history of the complaint, assessment of the pattern of breathing, and careful examination and auscultation will assist in determining the differential diagnoses for the cardiorespiratory problems
- It will also aid in selecting appropriate complementary exams, including thoracic radiography, echocardiography, arterial blood gas analysis, **electrocardiography** and **blood pressure measurement**

Equipment

- Stethoscope
- Stopwatch or timer

Patient preparation and positioning

- Assessment should be performed on the conscious animal.
- The patient should be standing if possible; this is particularly important for cardiac auscultation.
- Animals should be kept calm throughout the examination.

Observation

> **WARNING**
> - **Sternal recumbency, standing with elbows abducted and/or hyperventilating with the neck extended may indicate that the animal has dyspnoea.**

Body condition and shape

- In general, animals with airway-oriented diseases (tracheal collapse, chronic bronchitis, feline bronchial disease) will be in excellent systemic health and have a stable (or often increased) body condition score.
- Animals with parenchymal, pleural or cardiac disease with failure are more likely to be systemically debilitated or cachexic.
- Animals with congenital heart disease may have stunted growth.
- Obesity may be associated with lower airway disease in small breed dogs.
- Animals with chronic hyperpnoea can show barrel-chested changes.

Gait

- Cats with myocardial disease are at risk of systemic thromboembolism and may present with limb paresis.

Breathing pattern

- A visual appraisal of the respiratory pattern is made before the patient is stressed by an examination:
    - Restrictive respiratory diseases, such as pleural effusion and parenchymal disorders (pneumonia or oedema), cause rapid and shallow respiratory motions
    - Obstructive disorders, such as bronchitis, result in slow, deep breathing
    - Assessment of the phase of respiration that is predominantly affected (inspiratory *versus* expiratory) may help to localize obstructive disease:
        - Increased *expiratory* effort, prolonged expiratory time and abdominal effort on expiration should be considered suggestive of chronic lower airway disease
        - Increased *inspiratory* effort is suggestive of upper airway disease.

Physical examination

Mucous membrane colour

- Assess the colour of the mucous membranes:
    - Normal mucous membrane colour is pink to pale pink
    - *Pallor* can indicate anaemia, but can also be associated with severe peripheral vasoconstriction in low-output states or conditions of elevated sympathetic tone
    - *Cyanosis* indicates an increased concentration of desaturated haemoglobin, and ranges from slightly 'dusky' in mild cases to nearly navy blue in patients with severe hypoxaemia. Cyanosis is most often seen with severe hypoxaemia resulting from severe respiratory disease, congestive heart failure with pulmonary oedema or pleural effusion and right-to-left congenital shunts
    - Right-to-left (reversed) patent ductus arteriosus may result in differential cyanosis in which the cyanosis is only detected in the caudal half of the body
    - *Congested or Injected mucous membranes* occur with polycythaemia, systemic (toxaemia or septicaemia) or local inflammation, venous congestion, fever or exercise
    - *Cherry red* mucous membranes are seen in carbon monoxide toxicity.

Capillary refill time (CRT)

1 Apply pressure to the gum with a clean finger and then release.
2 This will cause blanching of the area.
3 The area should return to its normal colour within 1–2 seconds.

- An *increased CRT* (>2 seconds) indicates poor peripheral perfusion. Causes include low cardiac output, shock, dehydration or hypovolaemia.
- Patients in pain, with septic shock or with fever may demonstrate a *decreased CRT* (<1 second).

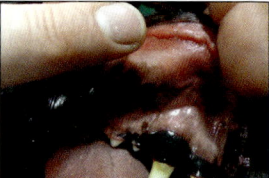

Jugular veins

- Visually inspect both jugular veins for distension and pulsation.
- In long-haired animals, it is possible to get an impression of jugular venous distension without clipping the hair if the coat is wetted with spirit.
- Jugular pulsation should not extend higher that one third of the neck in healthy standing dogs.

Distension

- In the absence of a cranial mediastinal mass or obstruction of the cranial vena cava, distension of the jugular veins indicates elevation of right atrial pressures.
- For animals with only a mild increase in right-sided pressure, compression of the cranial abdomen may increase venous return to the right heart sufficiently to cause temporary jugular distension ('hepatojugular reflux'). The distension resolves when the abdominal pressure is released.

Pulsation

- Jugular *pulsation* may be prominent with tricuspid regurgitation, pericardial disease, and when atrial contraction occurs against a non-compliant or restricted ventricle or a closed tricuspid valve during rhythm disturbances.

Peripheral pulse

- Suitable sites for monitoring the pulse include the following.

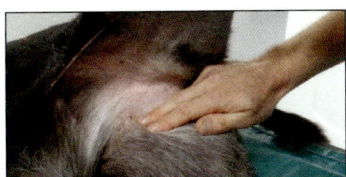

Femoral artery on medial aspect of femur

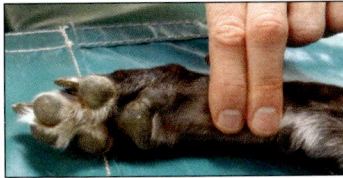

Digital artery on palmar aspect of carpus

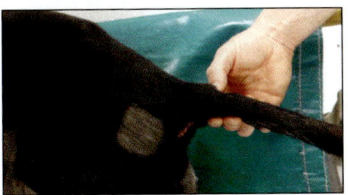

Coccygeal artery on ventral aspect of tail base

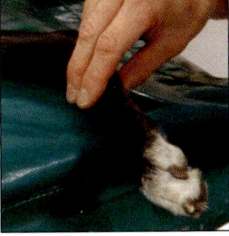

Dorsal pedal artery just distal to tarsus, between 2nd and 3rd metatarsals

1 Locate the artery with the fingertips.
2 Assess the pulse character, rate and rhythm.
3 Compare the pulse rate with the heart rate, preferably by simultaneous auscultation, to determine the presence of any pulse deficit.
4 Assess pulse on both sides for asymmetry.

- Weak pulses may reflect poor stroke volume or increased peripheral resistance.
- Strong pulses reflect an increased difference between diastolic and systolic pressure. Causes include: patent ductus arteriosus, severe aortic insufficiency and hyperthyroidism (cats).
- Detectable variations of the pulse quality with respiration (pulsus paradoxus) are usually associated with cardiac tamponade.
- Pulses may be absent or asymmetrical in patients with systemic thromboembolism.

Abdominal palpation

1 Assess the size of the liver:
   - Liver enlargement will accompany right-sided heart failure in dogs
   - The liver may be more palpable than usual in some cats with severe hyperpnoea and air trapping.
2 Assess the size of the kidneys:
   - Small, irregularly shaped kidneys may be associated with systemic hypertension
   - This should prompt **blood pressure measurement**.
3 Assess for the presence of abdominal effusion:
   - Small abdominal effusions may be appreciated as 'slipperiness' of the small intestines
   - Larger ascitic effusions are unmistakable on percussion of a fluid thrill.

Cardiac auscultation

Heart rate

- Heart rate can be helpful in differentiating cardiac from respiratory disease in dogs where respiratory disease is associated with elevated vagal tone, leading to an exaggerated respiratory sinus arrhythmia.
- Dogs with chronic heart failure are more likely to have increased sympathetic tone and an increased heart rate, although the degree of tachycardia may be modest.
- Care should be taken not to place too much reliance on heart rate in brachycephalic dogs with suspected heart failure, as concurrent airway obstruction may cause sufficient elevation in vagal tone that sinus arrhythmia persists despite overt heart failure.
- Cats do not always develop a consistent tachycardia with heart failure, and may be more likely than dogs to develop sinus bradycardia with life-threatening congestive failure signs.

Heart rhythm

- Normal dogs will have:
  - A regular heart rhythm
  - OR a sinus arrhythmia, where heart rate speeds up with inspiration and then slows with expiration.
- Cats normally have a regular heart rhythm.
- Bradyarrhythmias can be recognized by a slow heart rate.

- Atrial fibrillation sounds characteristically 'chaotic' on auscultation, but can still be confused with frequent atrial or ventricular premature beats.

Intensity of heart sounds

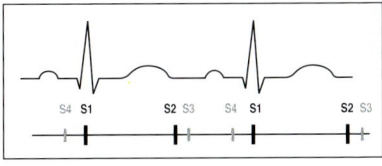

- Two heart sounds (S1 and S2) are normally heard in dogs and cats:
    - S1 occurs after closure of the atrioventricular valves, and is heard loudest at the apex of the heart
    - S2 occurs after closure of the aortic and pulmonic valves, and is heard loudest at the base of the heart.
- High cardiac output states, cardiac enlargement, thin body condition and increased sympathetic tone can *increase* the intensity of heart sounds.
- Pericardial effusion, severe myocardial failure, obesity, space-occupying lesions and pleural effusion may *decrease* intensity.
- Intensity may vary from beat to beat with rhythm disturbances including atrial fibrillation, frequent atrial or ventricular premature beats and irregular ventricular arrhythmia.

Additional heart sounds

- Additional heart sounds (S3 and S4) are associated with abnormal diastolic ventricular filling. These sounds are called *gallop sounds* and should not be audible in the normal dog or cat.
- Impaired ventricular relaxation can also cause an audible gallop, and may account for the presence of a gallop in some geriatric cats without obvious structural heart disease.
- In all other cats and dogs, a gallop sound can be considered to be a specific indication of heart disease.

Murmurs and clicks

- Murmurs are continuous sounds produced by turbulent blood flow:
    - They are more likely with high blood flow velocity (e.g. in pulmonic stenosis, aortic stenosis, mitral or tricuspid regurgitation)
    - Murmurs are characterized according to their timing, character, intensity and shape.

> **NOTES**
> - 'Flow' or physiological murmurs tend to be fairly quiet (<grade 2 or 3) and may vary in intensity.
> - They may occur with anaemia or can be normal in young animals.

- Systolic clicks are high-frequency transient heart sounds, usually associated with degenerative mitral valve disease.

Examination of the thoracic cavity

Thoracic palpation

1   Palpate the thorax for swellings, pain, rib fractures, subcutaneous emphysema or oedema.

2   Assess the strength of the apex beat using the fingers of one hand.

3   Determine the point of maximal intensity of the heart 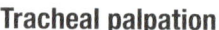 beat, using a stethoscope or fingers of one hand, to indicate any displacement by intrathoracic masses or effusion, and to detect any thrill (vibration of turbulence in blood flow). *This should preferably be done before auscultation.*

4   Using both hands, gently compress the thoracic cavity to assess for reduced compliance of the cranial thoracic cage, which could indicate a cranial mediastinal mass.

Tracheal palpation

■   Palpate the full length of the cervical trachea, using one hand, and observe for signs of sensitivity (usually indicated by a cough reflex).

■   Tracheal sensitivity is a non-specific sign of airway irritation and may be present in airway or parenchymal disease.

■   In dogs and cats with chronic bronchitis, airway collapse or pneumonia, a *harsh cough* is usually elicited with tracheal palpation.

■   A *soft cough* is more typical in dogs with pulmonary oedema.

Thoracic auscultation

1   Using a stethoscope, auscultate all lung fields on both sides of the thorax.

2   Note the presence, type and location of any abnormal lung sounds:

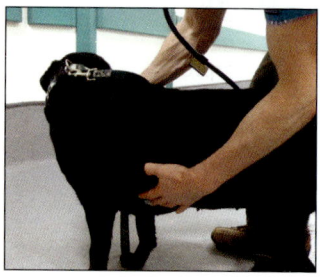

   ■   *Normal* sounds are termed bronchial, vesicular or bronchovesicular

   ■   *Crackles and wheezes* are examples of abnormal noises produced in diseased lungs

   ■   Determining the specific phase of the respiratory cycle in which abnormal lung sounds occur is important for categorizing the sound and determining the most likely pathology

- *Absence* of lung sounds is also an important finding:
  - It typically reflects disease of the pleural space
  - Consolidation of a lung segment can also lead to an absence of lung sounds
  - Loss of lung sounds *dorsally* generally indicates air accumulation
  - Loss of lung sounds *ventrally* indicates a pleural effusion or space-occupying mass.

Thoracic percussion

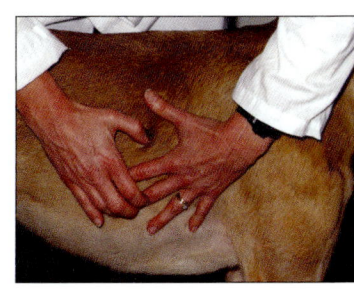

1 Place the fingers of one hand flat against the thoracic cage.
2 Curve the fingers of the other hand gently and hold them rigid.
3 Use the curved fingers of the free hand to strike the fingers on the chest wall, causing production of sounds.
4 Examine all lung fields to detect localized differences in sound transmission.

- Percussion causes vibration of the chest and intrathoracic structures, and the pitch reflects the underlying air-to-tissue ratio within the thorax.
- Over the heart, a dull percussive sound is heard because of the presence of soft tissue that dampens the transmission of sound.
- When the chest cavity is filled with fluid, or the lung is consolidated by disease, dull sounds are noted in the affected areas; whilst over air-filled lung structures, more resonant sounds are heard.
- In an animal with pneumothorax or air trapping, sounds have increased resonance.

FURTHER INFORMATION

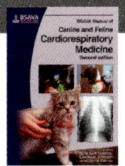

More detail on these procedures and interpretation of the results can be found in the *BSAVA Manual of Canine and Feline Cardiorespiratory Medicine*.

Dermatological examination

Whilst a complete history and thorough clinical examination are essential for dermatological cases, further diagnostic investigations are of paramount importance in reaching a definitive diagnosis. The following procedures can be performed in part, as required, or all together as part of a complete dermatological evaluation. (See also **Fine needle aspiration** and **Skin biopsy – punch biopsy**.)

Patient preparation and positioning

- The procedures below are usually performed in the conscious animal; a muzzle and/or sedation may be required for fractious patients.
- The patient may be positioned standing, sitting or in recumbency, depending on the area to be examined/sampled.
- An assistant may be required to hold the animal.
- **Adherence to good basic hygiene is required due to the possibility of infectious and zoonotic diseases.**

Initial examination

Equipment

- Good lighting
- Otoscope
- Magnifying glass or dermatoscope
- Camera

Technique

A systematic scrutiny of the animal from nose to tail tip is performed:

- It is important to examine the oral cavity, paws, ventrum and hindquarters
- A dermatoscope or magnifying glass allows detailed examination of lesions
- Otoscopy of both ear canals is performed
- Any deviations from normal skin, coat and mucosa are noted.
- Type and location of any lesions, both primary and secondary, are noted; photography can aid documentation.

Primary lesions
- Macule – non-palpable area of different colour, <1 cm diameter
- Patch – macule >1 cm diameter
- Papule – solid elevation <1 cm diameter
- Nodule – solid elevation >1 cm diameter
- Plaque – Platform-like elevation
- Vesicle – blister <1 cm, filled with clear fluid
- Bulla – blister >1 cm
- Pustule – vesicle filled with pus
- Tumour – large mass
- Wheal – raised, oedematous area (pitting on pressure)

continues ▶

continued ▶

Primary or secondary lesions

- Alopecia – loss of hair: spontaneous alopecia is primary; self-induced alopecia is secondary
- Scale – flakes of cornified cells
- Crust – dried exudate containing blood/serum/scales/pus
- Follicular casts – accumulation of keratin and follicular material like a sock around the base of the hair shaft
- Comedo – hair follicle plugged with keratin and sebum
- Hyperpigmentation – increased pigmentation
- Hypopigmentation – decreased pigmentation

Secondary lesions

- Collarette – circular, peeling lesion (often a remnant of a pustule)
- Scar – fibrous tissue replacing damaged dermis/subcutis
- Erosion – epidermal defect, not extending beneath the basement membrane
- Ulcer – skin defect below the level of the basement membrane
- Fissure – deep split
- Lichenification – thickening and hardening of the skin
- Excoriation – mild erosions caused by self-trauma

- A problem list is defined based on history, physical examination and initial dermatological examination.
- A differential diagnosis list for each problem is formulated in order to determine a diagnostic plan.

Organism suspected	Diagnostic tests
Bacteria	Cytology (swab, stain, oil immersion microscopy); culture and sensitivity testing; response to treatment
Dermatophytes	Wood's lamp; hair pluck; skin scrape; fungal culture
Malassezia yeast	Cytology; tape strip; fungal culture; response to treatment
Fleas	Macroscopic examination; coat brushing; response to treatment
Ticks	Macroscopic examination
Lice	Macroscopic examination; coat brushing
Cheyletiella mites	Tape strip; skin scrape
Demodex mites	Skin scrape (deep); hair pluck; impression smear of pustule; skin biopsy
Sarcoptes/Notoedres mites	Skin scrape (deep); serology; skin biopsy; response to treatment
Otodectes mites	Cotton swab of ear cerumen
Trombicula mites	Tape strip

Wood's lamp examination

To check for dermatophytosis.

Equipment

- Wood's lamp
- Magnifying glass

Technique

1 Switch on the Wood's lamp and allow it to warm up for 5–10 minutes.
2 The animal should be placed in a darkened room.
3 Examine the hair coat with the Wood's lamp. A magnifying glass may also be used.
4 Observe for bright apple-green fluorescence of hairs; 5 minutes should be spent looking, as the fluorescence is sometimes delayed.

> **NOTES**
>
> - Unfortunately, not all strains of *Microsporum canis* fluoresce, the number showing positive fluorescence varying between 30 and 90% in published reports.
> - Other less common dermatophytes that may also induce fluorescence include *M. distortum*, *M. audouinii*, *M. equinum* and *Trichophyton schoenleinii*.
> - False positive fluorescence may be observed due to certain topical medications, dead skin scales and some bacteria.

Coat brushing for fleas

Equipment

- Flea comb or stiff plastic hair brush
- White paper
- Container, such as a Petri dish
- Hand lens
- Microscope, slides and cover slips

Technique

1 With the patient standing on a sheet of white paper, brush the coat over several minutes to collect surface debris using a flea comb or stiff plastic hairbrush.
2 Collect the debris into a container, such as a Petri dish, and examine with a hand lens.
3 Transfer the material on to microscope slides and examine.

Wet paper test

The patient can either be brushed while standing on dampened white paper OR debris collected on dry paper can be dampened with damp cotton wool. Black flea faeces give a reddish brown stain on the damp paper or cotton wool.

Coat brushing for dermatophytes: Mackenzie toothbrush technique

Equipment

- New or sterilized toothbrush
- Fungal culture medium

Technique

1   Brush the **whole coat** of the animal with a new or sterilized toothbrush for several minutes. It is helpful to brush against the natural flow of hairs.
2   Touch the toothbrush head on to a fungal culture plate several times and incubate as per the manufacturer's instructions.

Hair plucks

Primarily to assess hair structure and to check for ectoparasites and dermatophytes associated with the hair root.

Equipment

- Haemostats
- Microscope slides or coverslips
- Clear adhesive tape
- Liquid paraffin (mineral oil)
- Microscope
- ± Fungal culture medium

Technique

1   Pluck several hairs, including the roots, using the haemostats.
2   Place the hairs on to a piece of clear adhesive tape and affix this to a microscope slide, or mount under a coverslip in liquid paraffin.
3   Examine under a microscope:
    - Examine the tips of the hairs for evidence of breaking and damage, indicated by abrupt, blunt or frayed ends instead of the tapering tips of normal hairs
    - Examine the roots to assess whether hairs are in anagen (a pronounced bulb present) or telogen (club root with barbs or frayed appearance) phase
    - The presence of comedones or follicular plugs can also be detected, surrounding the shafts towards the root end of plucked hairs
    - Examination of the roots of plucked hairs may reveal the presence of *Demodex* or *Cheyletiella* mites, louse eggs or fungal spores (dermatophytosis).
4   Hairs can also be placed on to fungal culture medium and incubated as per the manufacturer's instructions.

Adhesive tape impressions

Primarily for cytological examination of the skin surface, but also to check for ectoparasites.

Equipment

- Clippers
- Microscope slides
- Clear adhesive tape
- Stain such as Diff-Quik
- Microscope

Technique

1. Firmly press a piece of clear adhesive tape against an unhaired (or clipped) region of skin.
2. Attach both ends of the tape to a slide, leaving the middle portion free.
3. Stain the tape strip with Diff-Quik or equivalent. Gently rinse off excess stain. Detach one end of the tape and stick the whole strip down flat on the slide.
4. Blot off excess liquid and perform cytological examination of the tape using a microscope.
5. *Alternatively,* the tape strip can be examined unstained for ectoparasites.

Smears of expressed follicular contents

Primarily to check for ectoparasites.

Equipment

- Microscope slides and coverslips
- Liquid paraffin (mineral oil)
- No. 10 scalpel
- Microscope

Technique

1. Squeeze the skin to extrude material from hair follicles.
2. Draw a clean microscope slide across the surface to smear this material on to the slide. *Alternatively,* material may be collected on a scalpel blade and then transferred to a slide.
3. No staining is necessary, although a little liquid paraffin may be used for coverslip mounting.
4. Examine the slide with a microscope for ectoparasites, especially *Demodex* mites.

Smears of aural wax/exudate

Primarily for cytological examination and to check for ectoparasites.

Equipment

- Microscope slides and coverslips
- Liquid paraffin (mineral oil)

- Cotton bud
- Microscope
- ± Stain such as Diff-Quik

Technique

1 Collect debris from external ear canal using a cotton bud.
2 Smear debris onto a microscope slide.
3 Liquid paraffin may be used to disperse the sample and for coverslip mounting.
4 Examine the slide unstained with a microscope for ear mites and their eggs.
5 Slides can be stained for cytological examination with a microscope.

Skin scrape

Primarily to check for ectoparasites, but may also identify dermatophytosis.

Equipment

- Clippers
- Saline or mounting medium
- No. 10 scalpel blade (blunted)
- Microscope slides and coverslips
- Liquid paraffin (mineral oil)
- 10% potassium hydroxide
- Blue–black ink or lactophenol cotton blue
- Microscope

Technique

1 Clip overlying hair.
2 The skin can be moistened with a drop of mounting medium or saline.
3 Squeeze the skin between the fingers.
4 Gently scrape the top layer of the skin surface until capillary oozing of blood occurs, and transfer the sample to a microscope slide.

> **NOTES**
>
> - For sarcoptic mange: take superficial scrapes from primary lesions (papules and crusts) at the edges of areas with lesion; avoid ulcerated areas.
> - For *Demodex* mites: take deep scrapes from areas with comedones.
> - For dermatophyte infections: sample the advancing edge of new lesions to include hair and skin scale.

5 Apply a drop of liquid paraffin or potassium hydroxide to the sample on the slide.

> **NOTES**
>
> - Liquid paraffin allows immediate examination of slides and identification of live mites, but has the disadvantage of not clearing debris.
> - 10% potassium hydroxide allows good separation of keratinocytes and clearing of material, but is caustic to skin itself and kills mites.
> - 10% potassium hydroxide is preferred for identification of fungal elements.

6 Place a coverslip over the sample and mounting medium, and examine with a microscope under low and then high power.

7 The addition of a drop of blue–black ink or lactophenol cotton blue may permit fungal structures to be seen more easily.

Stained smears from pustules or lesions

Primarily for cytological examination. Occasionally, ectoparasites such as *Demodex* mites may also be seen. (See also **Fine needle aspiration**)

Equipment

- Hypodermic needles: 21 G
- Microscope slides and coverslips
- Stain such as Diff-Quik
- Microscope

Technique

1 Rupture an intact pustule with a sterile hypodermic needle, and smear its contents on to a clean microscope slide.

2 Impression smears can also be made from ulcerated lesions or the cut surface of excised lesions.

3 Air-dry the slide.

4 Stain with Diff-Quik or equivalent, according to the manufacturer's instructions.

5 Perform cytological evaluation using a microscope.

Culture of microorganisms – bacteria

- *Sterile* swabs and bacterial transport medium are required.
- Samples for bacterial culture should be taken from new lesions or recently ruptured pustules or vesicles and *not* from old, crusted or excoriated lesions.
- **Do not use any aseptic skin preparation or surgical spirit before sampling.**
- Rupture an intact pustule with a sterile needle and absorb the contents on to a sterile swab. Place the swab into transport medium before sending samples to the laboratory.
- *Alternatively,* tissue from a **skin biopsy** may be submitted in a sterile container for bacterial culture.

Culture of microorganisms – fungi

- Samples can be obtained from coat brushings or hair plucks (see earlier).
- Submission of a sample to an external reference diagnostic laboratory for fungal culture is preferable. Consult the external laboratory for their packaging requirements/recommendations.
- Samples can be cultured in house on Sabouraud's dextrose agar in Petri dishes. Incubate in a temperature-controlled environment, or at room temperature in the UK. Examine plates twice weekly for up to 3–4 weeks. This gives good results, allowing clear identification of fungal colony morphology and fungal elements.
- Samples can be cultured in house on DTM (dermatophyte test medium). This is prone to false negative and false positive results, however, and is no longer recommended.

Neurological examination

Indications/Use

- To diagnose and localize disorders of the nervous system
- To provide information on the severity of some disorders

Equipment

- Reflex hammer
- A bright light source
- Cotton bud dampened with sterile saline
- Artery forceps
- 70% surgical spirit
- Food (with potent smell)
- Ball of cotton wool

Patient preparation and positioning

- The neurological examination should be performed with the animal conscious and without the administration of any sedation.
- Animals should be kept calm throughout the examination.
- Positioning will vary, depending on the part of the examination being performed.

Observation

The following parameters should be observed before starting the 'hands-on' part of the examination:

- Mental status and behaviour
- Posture and body position at rest
- Gait (see **Orthopaedic examination**)
- Abnormal involuntary movements.

Cranial nerve assessment

Olfactory nerve – CN I

- Smell is assessed by testing the animal's response (sniffing or licking of the nose, aversion of the head) to aromatic substances (e.g. surgical spirit) whilst it is blindfolded or has its eyes covered. Care should be taken not to use irritating substances that could stimulate the trigeminal nerve and cause similar responses. *Alternatively,* the animal's response to food can be observed, again whilst it is blindfolded or has its eyes covered.

Optic nerve – CN II

- Vision tests are described in **Ophthalmic examination**.

Oculomotor nerve – CN III

1 Observe eye position and movements (a) at rest and (b) by testing for normal physiological nystagmus (vestibulo-ocular reflex), by moving the head from side to side as well as up

and down (see Vestibulocochlear nerve – CN VIII, below).

- Normal physiological nystagmus (also called 'jerk' nystagmus) is an involuntary rhythmic movement of the eyes, which typically presents with a slow phase in one direction and a quick phase in the other direction. Dysfunction of CN III will result in a resting ventrolateral strabismus and inability to move the eyeball medially during physiological nystagmus testing. Ptosis of the upper eyelid also occurs with dysfunction of CN III.

2 The *parasympathetic* function of CN III can be assessed by observation of pupil size and evaluation of the pupillary light reflex (PLR; see **Ophthalmic examination**). Lesions will result in mydriasis of the affected eye. The PLR tests the integrity of the retina, optic nerve, optic tract, lateral geniculate nucleus, oculomotor nucleus, CN III and pupillary muscle.

Trochlear nerve – CN IV

- Eye position at rest is observed. Lesions of the trochlear nerve produce a dorsolateral strabismus (extorsion) of the contralateral eye.

Trigeminal nerve – CN V

Photos from *BSAVA Manual of Canine and Feline Neurology* and courtesy of Laurent Garosi

- The *motor* function of CN V is assessed by evaluating the size and symmetry of the masticatory muscles and testing the resistance of the jaw to opening the mouth.

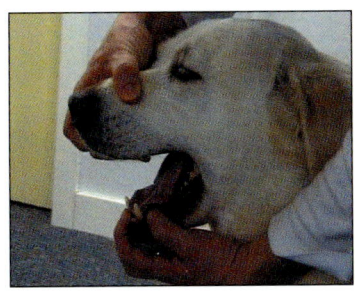

- The *sensory* function (sensation of the face) can be individually tested by:
  - **i** The corneal reflex observed on touching the cornea with a damp cotton bud (ophthalmic branch)
  - **ii** The palpebral reflex observed on touching the medial or lateral canthus of the eye (ophthalmic or maxillary branch, respectively)

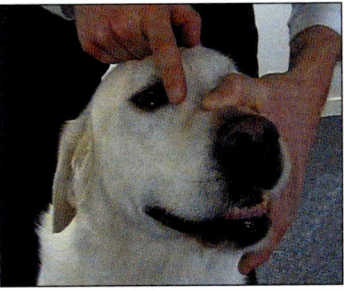

   iii   The response to stimulation of the nasal mucosa (ophthalmic branch).

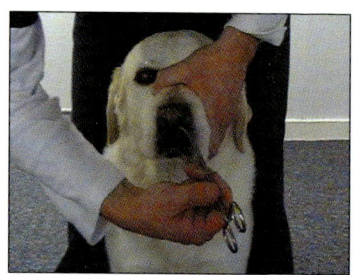

- A reflex response is best distinguished from a conscious response by stimulating the nasal mucosa: the normal animal will pull its head away, while the animal with forebrain disease may blink or show a facial twitch, but not show a conscious reaction.

Abducent nerve – CN VI

1 Observe the eye position and movement at rest.
2 Test for normal physiological nystagmus (see above).
3 Test for normal eyeball retraction during the corneal reflex.
   - Lesions of the abducent nerve result in: an ipsilateral convergent medial strabismus; an inability to move the eyeball laterally when evaluating the horizontal physiological nystagmus; and an inability to retract the eyeball.

Facial nerve – CN VII

1 The *motor* function of CN VII is primarily assessed by observation of the face for symmetry (position of the ears and lip commissure on each side within the same plane, symmetry of the palpebral fissure), spontaneous blinking and movement of the nostrils. Motor dysfunction produces: ipsilateral drooping of and inability to move the ear and lip; widened palpebral fissure and absent spontaneous and provoked blinking; absent abduction of the nostril during inspiration; and 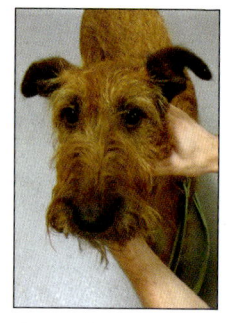 deviation of the nose toward the normal side due to the unopposed muscle tone on the unaffected side.
2 The **Schirmer tear test** (see **Ophthalmic examination**) can evaluate the *parasympathetic* supply of the lacrimal gland associated with CN VII. Examining the mouth for moist mucosa can subjectively assess salivation. Also assess the nose for dryness (xeromycteria), as this can result from disruption to the parasympathetic supply of the lateral nose glands via CN VII.

Vestibulocochlear nerve – CN VIII

1 Observe the animal's body and head posture at rest, and evaluate its gait (see **Orthopaedic examination**). This function can also be more specifically assessed by testing the *vestibulo-ocular reflex* (see above). Vestibular dysfunction may result in

any or all of the following: head tilt; falling; leaning; rolling; circling; abnormal spontaneous and/or positional nystagmus; positional strabismus; and ataxia.

2 The *auditory* function of CN VIII is difficult to assess. The startle reaction consists of observing the animal's response to noise (e.g. handclap, whistle), but this does not detect unilateral or partial deafness. The best assessment is the animal's response to noise when asleep: most owners can report whether they have to touch their animal in order to wake them. Electrophysiological assessment is necessary to confirm and assess the severity of the hearing loss.

Glossopharyngeal and vagus nerves – CN IX and CN X

- The *pharyngeal* (swallowing or gag) reflex can be evaluated by:
  - **i** Applying external pressure to the hyoid bones to stimulate swallowing
  - **ii** Stimulating the pharynx with a finger to elicit a gag reflex
  - **iii** Watching the animal eat or drink
  - **iv** Opening the animal's mouth wide.
- CN IX dysfunction results in dysphagia, absent gag reflex and reduced pharyngeal tone if deficits are bilateral.
- CN X dysfunction results in dysphagia, inspiratory dyspnoea (due to laryngeal paralysis), voice changes (dysphonia) and regurgitation (due to megaoesophagus in the case of bilateral vagal disorder).

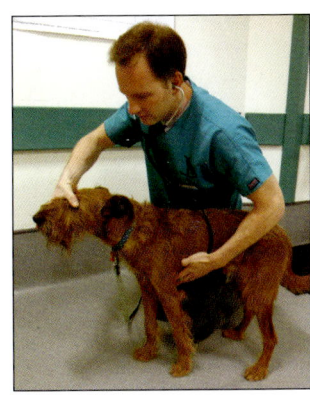

- The *parasympathetic* portion of CN X can be evaluated by testing the oculocardiac reflex. This is achieved by applying digital pressure to both eyeballs and observing simultaneously a reflex bradycardia (also mediated by CN V).

Accessory nerve – CN XI

- Lesions of this nerve result in atrophy of the trapezius muscle. Observe the position of the neck, as this may be deviated toward the affected side in chronic cases. Isolated lesions of the accessory nerve are an extremely rare finding.

Hypoglossal nerve – CN XII

1 Inspect the tongue for atrophy, asymmetry or deviation to one side.

2 Manually stretching the tongue and observing a voluntary retraction assesses the tongue's tone.

3 Applying food paste to the nose and observing the animal licking assesses the tongue's movement.
  - Lesions affecting CN XII can result in problems with prehension, mastication and deglutition.

Postural reaction testing

Photos from *BSAVA Manual of Canine and Feline Neurology* and courtesy of Laurent Garosi

Paw placement

1 Sequentially place each paw in an abnormal position (turned over so that the dorsal surface is in contact with the ground) and determine how quickly the animal corrects it. The animal should be standing squarely on all four limbs, with the majority of its weight supported by an assistant.

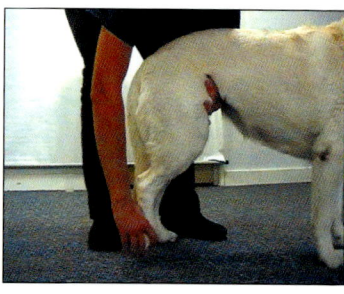

2 Place a piece of paper under a weight-bearing foot and pull it slowly in a lateral direction. A normal response is to pick up the limb and replace it in the correct position. Repeat with the other feet in turn.

Hopping reaction

- The hopping reaction is tested by holding the animal so that the majority of its weight is placed on one limb while the animal is moved laterally. Normal animals hop on the tested limb to accommodate a new body position as their centre of gravity is displaced laterally. The hop should be initiated as the shoulder or hip moves lateral to the paw, and the animal then replaces the limb appropriately under the newly positioned body. An equal response should be seen on both sides.

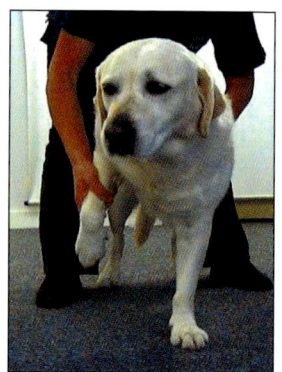

Placing response

- Non-visual:
  - iii. Cover the animal's eyes.
  - iv. Lift the animal until the distal part of the thoracic limb is brought into contact with the edge of a table.
  - v. The normal response is for the animal immediately to place its foot on the table surface.
- Visual placing:
  - i. Allow the animal to see the table surface.
  - ii. Lift the animal toward the edge of the table.
  - iii. Normal animals will reach for the surface before the paw touches the table.

Hemi-walking and wheelbarrowing

- Hemi-walking:
    - Tests the ability of the animal to walk on the thoracic and pelvic limbs of one side of the body, while you are holding the limbs on the other side
    - i   Push the animal away from the side on which its limbs are supported
    - ii Assess the speed and coordination of movements that restore the appropriate limb position in response to the change in body position.
- Wheelbarrowing:
    - Tests the thoracic limbs; highlights subtle weakness and ataxia
    - i   Lift the pelvic limbs off the ground by supporting the animal under the abdomen
    - ii Force the animal to walk forwards.

Spinal reflexes: muscle tone and size

Spinal reflex evaluation is performed to classify the neurological disorder as being of LMN or UMN type. This allows the examiner to localize the lesion to specific spinal cord segments or peripheral nerves. Spinal reflexes are best tested with the animal relaxed in lateral recumbency, with the side to be tested uppermost.

- *Lower motor neuron:* If LMNs are damaged, the following clinical signs are characteristically found:
    - Flaccid paresis and/or paralysis
    - Reduced or absent reflexes
    - Reduced or absent muscle tone
    - Early and severe muscle atrophy.
- *Upper motor neuron:* If UMNs are damaged, the following clinical signs are characteristically found:
    - Spastic paresis and/or paralysis
    - Normal to increased reflex activity (hyperreflexia)
    - Increased extensor muscle tone (hypertonia) manifested as a resistance to passive manipulation of the limbs
    - Chronic mild to moderate muscle atrophy (disuse atrophy).

Thoracic limbs

Withdrawal (flexor) reflex

This evaluates the integrity of spinal cord segments C6–T2 (and associated nerve roots) as well as the brachial plexus and peripheral nerves.

> **NOTES**
>
> - The withdrawal reflex in the thoracic or pelvic limbs does *not* depend on the animal's *conscious* perception of noxious stimuli (nociceptive function).
> - The withdrawal reflex is a segmental spinal cord reflex that depends only on the function of the local spinal cord segments.

1   With the animal in lateral recumbency, apply a noxious stimulus by pinching the nailbed or digit with the fingers or artery forceps.
2   This stimulus causes a reflex contraction of the flexor muscles and withdrawal of the tested limb.
3   If this withdrawal reflex is absent, test individual toes to detect whether specific nerve deficits are present.
4   When testing the flexor reflex, observe the contralateral limb for extension (crossed-extensor reflex), indicating a UMN lesion cranial to the C6 spinal cord segment.

Extensor carpi radialis reflex

- This evaluates the integrity of spinal cord segments C7–T2 and associated nerve roots as well as the radial nerve.
1   Strike the extensor carpi radialis muscle belly with a reflex hammer along the craniolateral aspect of the proximal antebrachium.
2   The desired reaction is a slight extension of the carpus.

Pelvic limbs

Photos from *BSAVA Manual of Canine and Feline Neurology* and courtesy of Laurent Garosi

Withdrawal (flexor) reflex

This evaluates the integrity of spinal cord segments L4–S2 (and associated nerve roots) as well as the femoral and sciatic nerves.

> **NOTES**
> - The withdrawal reflex in the thoracic or pelvic limbs does *not* depend on the animal's *conscious* perception of noxious stimuli (nociceptive function).
> - The withdrawal reflex is a segmental spinal cord reflex that only depends on the function of the local spinal cord segments.

1   With the animal in lateral recumbency, apply a noxious stimulus by pinching the nailbed or digit with the fingers or artery forceps.
2   This stimulus causes a reflex contraction of the flexor muscles and withdrawal of the tested limb.
3   A normal reflex constitutes flexion of the hip (femoral nerve function), stifle and hock (sciatic nerve function).
4   The hock must be extended in order to evaluate sciatic function (i.e. hock flexion).
5   A crossed-extensor reflex in the pelvic limb indicates a UMN lesion cranial to the L4 spinal cord segment.

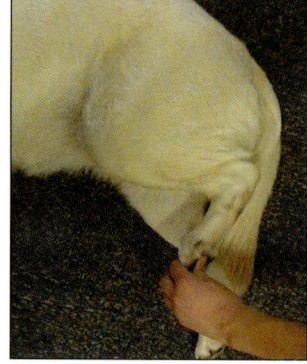

Patellar reflex

This evaluates the integrity of spinal cord segments L4–L6 (and associated nerve roots) as well as the femoral nerve.

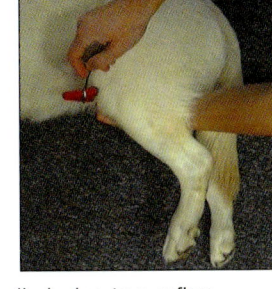

1 The animal is placed in lateral recumbency, with the stifle slightly flexed and the tested limb supported by placing one hand under the thigh.
2 Striking the patellar tendon with a reflex hammer induces extension of the limb due to a reflex contraction of the quadriceps femoris muscle.
3 A weak or absent reflex indicates a lesion of the L4–L6 spinal cord segments or the femoral nerve.

Evaluation of the tail and anus

Perineal reflex

Stimulation of the perineum with artery forceps should result in contraction of the anal sphincter, and flexion of the tail.

Sensory evaluation

Photos from *BSAVA Manual of Canine and Feline Neurology* and courtesy of Laurent Garosi

Cutaneous trunci (panniculus) reflex

1 Place the animal in sternal recumbency or in a standing position.
2 Pinch the skin of the dorsal trunk with artery forceps between vertebral level T2 and L4–L5, and observe for a contraction of the cutaneous trunci muscles bilaterally, producing a twitch of the overlying skin.
3 The reflex is present in the thoracolumbar region and absent in the neck and sacral region.
4 Testing is begun at the level of the ilial wings: if the reflex is present at this level the entire pathway is intact and further testing is not necessary.
5 With spinal cord lesions, this reflex is lost caudal to the spinal cord segment affected, indicating the presence of a transverse myelopathy. Pinching the skin cranial to the lesion results in a normal reflex, while stimulation of the skin caudal to the lesion does not elicit any reflex.

Deep pain perception

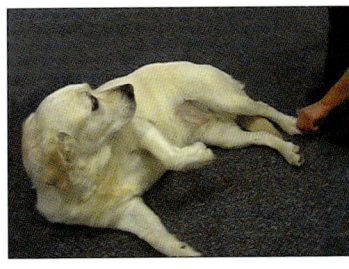

1 Place the animal on its side, ideally with a second person talking to or stroking it to distract attention.
2 Apply an initial gentle squeeze to the digits to elicit the withdrawal reflex.

3 If the animal does not manifest any behavioural response following a gentle squeeze, apply heavy pressure to the bones of the digits with artery forceps.

4 Only a severe bilateral spinal cord lesion impairs the conscious perception of deep pain. For this reason, testing of deep pain perception is a useful prognostic indicator in cases of spinal cord disease.

5 This conscious pain perception must be assessed in all limbs and/or the tail that are determined to have no voluntary movements (paralysis/plegia). Testing of deep pain perception is **not required** in limbs for which there is visible voluntary motor function.

6 The expected reaction is a behavioural response such as turning the head, trying to bite or vocalization, or a physiological response to perception of pain such as an increase in heart rate or pupil dilation. **Withdrawal of the limb is only the flexor reflex and should not be taken as evidence of pain sensation.**

Spinal palpation and neck manipulation

Photos from *BSAVA Manual of Canine and Feline Neurology* and courtesy of Laurent Garosi

■ Spinal palpation and neck manipulation to assess for pain should *only* be performed at the end of the neurological examination.

1 Using the fingers of one hand, apply firm pressure to the thoracic and lumbar spine whilst observing for a pain response.

2 The neck should be manipulated in dorsal, ventral and both lateral directions, whilst observing for a pain response.

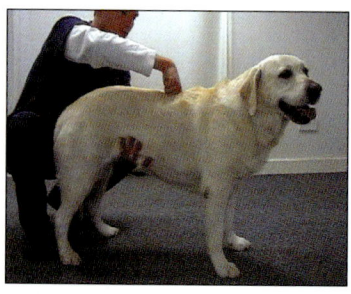 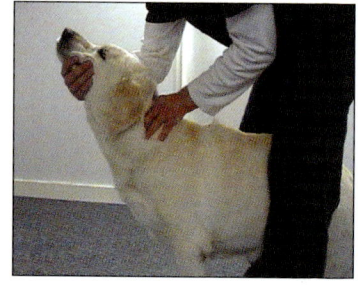

FURTHER INFORMATION

More detail on these procedures and interpretation of the results can be found in the *BSAVA Manual of Canine and Feline Neurology.*

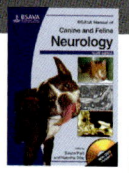

Ophthalmic examination

Indications/Use

- Suspected primary ocular disease
- As part of investigations for suspected or confirmed neurological disease
- As part of investigations for suspected or confirmed systemic diseases with possible ocular involvement, e.g. hypertension, diabetes, lymphoma

Equipment

- Bright focal light source, such as a Finoff transilluminator
- Schirmer tear test strips
- Stop watch
- Direct ophthalmoscope
- Mydriatic – 1% tropicamide
- Ophthalmic lens – 28–30 dioptres (D)
- Topical local anaesthetic – 0.5% proxymetacaine eyedrops
- A goniolens and sterile lubricant (viscous tears, e.g. 1% Celluvisc or sterile K–Y Jelly)
- Applanation or rebound tonometer (e.g. TonoPen, TonoPen Vet)
- Fluorescein test strips (or multi-use fluorescein vials; NB these should only be used once) and cobalt blue light source
- 0.9% sterile saline and 5 ml syringe
- Soft paper towel
- Cytobrush and glass slides

Patient preparation and position

- The ophthalmic examination should be performed on the conscious animal without sedation. A muzzle should be used if required.
- Position the animal in a standing or sitting position, on a table if possible.
- An assistant is required for restraint and should support the head in a fixed position by holding the animal underneath the chin.

The ophthalmic examination

Hands-off examination

1 Assess for evidence of pain: tears, increased blinking, blepharospasm, photophobia.
2 Assess orbital and periocular conformation, globe size and position. Check for asymmetry or strabismus.
3 Check the following reflexes:
   i Vestibulo-ocular reflex: Reflex eye movements normally allow stabilization of an image on the retina, resulting in slow eye movements opposite to the direction of head movement
   ii Menace response: Direction of a splayed hand towards the eye should elicit a blink or retraction of the head. Avoid creating a draught of air directed towards the cornea.

4   Examine the conformation of the upper and lower eyelids and the position of the nictitating membrane.
5   Note the presence and nature of any ocular discharge.
6   An **obstacle course** may be improvised from chairs, waste bins, etc. The animal's performance should be assessed: for both eyes; with one eye covered; and in bright and dim lighting conditions.

Schirmer tear test I (STT I)

The STT I measures *aqueous production* in the un-anaesthetized eye and is an indicator of basal and reflex tear production.

> **NOTE**
>
> Perform STT I before manipulation of the eyelids or direct application of light sources to the eyes, as these may falsely elevate test results.

Technique

1   The test strips are notched near one end: identify the notched end of the test strip while it is still in its packet.
2   Bend the test strip transversely at the level of the notch.
3   Remove the test strip from the packet, only handling the end away from the notch.
4   Evert the lateral lower eyelid and place the notched end of the strip in the lateral half of the lower conjunctival sac, so that the notch is at the level of the lid margin and the strip is in contact with the lower lid and cornea.
5   Release the test strip and the eyelid and hold the lids closed, retaining the test strip securely in position.
6   After 1 minute remove the test strip from the eye.
7   Record the distance aqueous tears have travelled from the notch, indicated by the blue dye.

Test results

- Dogs: Mean reference value = 20 mm/min; <15mm/min is suggestive of keratoconjunctivitis sicca (KCS)
- Cats: Mean reference value = 17 mm/min

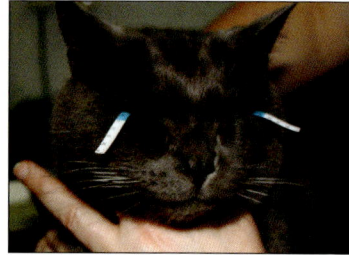

Pupillary light reflexes

1   Note pupil size in normal room light.
2   Continue in a dimly lit room.
3   Direct a bright light axially through the pupil in each eye. Look for constriction of the pupil in response to direct light and light directed at the contralateral eye.

4 In the 'swinging flashlight test', the light is directed at each eye alternately, with the observer noting the direct (in the same eye) and indirect (in the other eye) responses.

Eyelids and conjunctiva

1 Retract the upper eyelid and examine the dorsal bulbar conjunctiva; evert the lid margin and check the upper palpebral conjunctiva and upper lacrimal punctum.

2 Apply pressure to the globe through the upper lid and protrude the nictitating membrane, checking its leading edge, its alignment and its outer surface.

3 Retract the lower lid and assess the conjunctiva, and the lower lacrimal punctum as it enters the fornix.

Cornea

1 Check the corneal (Purkinje) reflex (the smoothness and sharpness of the reflection of a light on the corneal surface).

2 Examine the cornea. Check for irregularities, opacities, vascularization and pigmentation.

Anterior chamber

1 Direct a bright focal light source into the anterior chamber from various angles and observe from various angles.

2 Note the depth of the anterior chamber and any abnormal contents.

3 Examine the iris, pupil margin and lens.

Distant direct ophthalmoscopy

The room should be darkened, but mydriatic drops are not required. The examination is conducted at arm's length.

1 Set the ophthalmoscope to the operator's neutral setting (see instrument manual for instructions).

2 Find the tapetal reflex (the green or yellow light reflected from the tapetum) by looking into the pupil horizontally or slightly upwards. Any genuine opacity, such as cataracts, corneal and vitreous opacities, in the path of the tapetal reflex will obscure it and appear black.

3 Lesions can be roughly *localized* in an anteroposterior direction, by taking advantage of the effect of parallax: as the observer moves to one side, the opacity may also appear to move. The direction of this movement can give an indication as to the location of the opacity:

■ Opacities anterior to the plane of the pupil will appear to move in the opposite direction

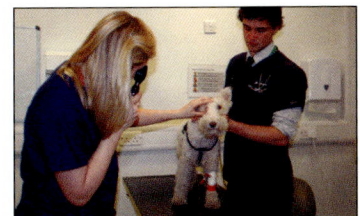

■ Opacities in the plane of the pupil (i.e. anterior cataracts), will remain in the same position.

Close direct ophthalmoscopy

The direct ophthalmoscope is used to examine the fundus. The image is upright and highly magnified, but the field of view is very narrow.

1 Dilate the pupils with 1–2 drops of 1% tropicamide solution per eye. Mydriasis occurs in 15–20 minutes and lasts for 6 hours.
2 Set the ophthalmoscope to the operator's neutral setting (see instrument manual for instructions).
3 Hold the ophthalmoscope vertically, with it touching your own orbital margin. Be close to the patient's eye, so as to maximize the field of view and eliminate distractions such as the iris.
4 Find the optic disc: this is more or less at the posterior pole. Evaluate the disc for size, swelling, colour, blood vessels, etc.
5 Make a systematic examination of the fundus by examining it in quarters. Evaluate the retina for normal variation or changes in colour, reflectivity, pigment, haemorrhage, oedema and detachment.
6 Focus back through to the anterior eye. Exact dioptre settings required for this depend on the presence or absence of vitreal abnormalities and the distance of the ophthalmoscope from the patient's eye.
  - +10 D to +15 D is usually required to bring the lens into focus.
  - +15 D to +20 D is required to examine structures anterior to the lens.

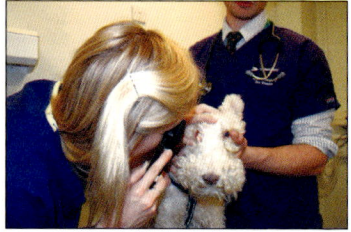

Indirect ophthalmoscopy

When compared to direct ophthalmoscopy, indirect methods give an inverted, reversed image which is less highly magnified but covers a much wider angle of view.

1 Dilate the pupils with 1–2 drops of 1% tropicamide solution per eye. Mydriasis occurs in 15–20 minutes and lasts for 6 hours.
2 Hold an ophthalmic lens (28–30 D) between your index finger and thumb, with the more convex side of the lens facing you.
3 Rest your hand on the patient's head, to allow you to position the lens stably in front of the patient's eye, but initially hold the lens away from the patient's eye.
4 Hold a bright light source (Finoff transilluminator) against your temple and align your eye, the light source and the patient's pupil along the same axis. Correct alignment will result in visualization of a tapetal reflection.
5 Insert the lens in front of the patient's eye to examine the fundus. If the image of the fundus is lost, repeat steps 2–4.

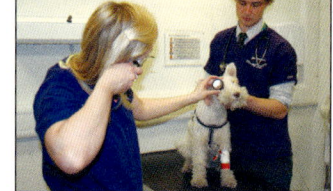

Ancillary tests

These are performed as required for the individual case.

Gonioscopy

Gonioscopy is the examination of the iridocorneal angle and ciliary cleft. It is indicated for cases of suspected glaucoma.

> **NOTE**
>
> Gonioscopy should be performed *prior to* pharmacological dilation of the pupil.

1 Apply 1–2 drops of 0.5% proxymetacaine to the cornea. This will be effective in 1 minute and the effect will last for 10–20 minutes.
2 Apply sterile lubricant to the concave side of the inverted goniolens. Air bubbles should be avoided, because they will distort light and prevent adequate visualization.
3 Place the goniolens on to the cornea in one quick motion so as not to lose the lubricant.
4 Using a bright light source, such as a direct ophthalmoscope, examine the entire iridocorneal angle and ciliary cleft systematically.

Tonometry

Tonometry is the indirect measurement of intraocular pressure (IOP). Where possible, this should be performed as part of the routine ophthalmic examination. It is specifically indicated for cases of suspected glaucoma. Various methods can be used, including rebound and applanation techniques.

Applanation tonometry using a TonoPen

1 Apply 1–2 drops of 0.5% proxymetacaine to the cornea. This will be effective in 1 minute and the effect will last 10–20 minutes.
2 Restrain the patient with its head and eyes directed forwards and its eyelids held open against the orbital rim. *Care must be taken not to press against the globe, because this might falsely elevate the IOP.*
3 Place a disposable sterile protective sheath over the tip of the TonoPen.
4 Using the probe tip, gently and repeatedly contact the central area of the cornea.
5 Record the IOP measurement from the digital screen at the sound of the longer beep.

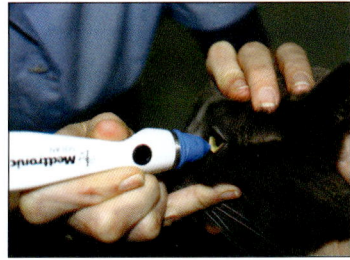

Rebound tonometry using a TonoPen Vet

1 Topical anaesthesia is not required

2 Restrain the patient with the head and eyes directed forwards and the eyelids held open against the orbital rim. *Care must be taken not to press against the globe, because this might falsely elevate the IOP.*

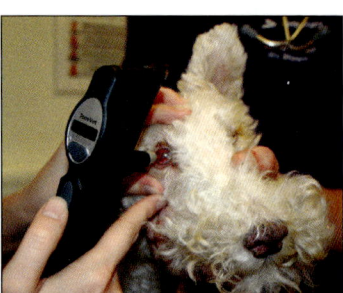

3 Read the manufacturer's instructions and correctly turn on, load and calibrate the instrument for the species you are dealing with.

4 Press the button six times; the probe will exit the machine and touch the cornea. At the long beep, the reading will be displayed and this should be recorded.

Fluorescein test

The fluorescein test is indicated for diagnosis of corneal ulcers, where epithelium is absent and the stroma is exposed. Note that fluorescein will not stain healed ulcers that have re-epithelialized or Descemet's membrane.

1 Use a 5 ml syringe to wet the test strip thoroughly with sterile saline.

2 Touch the test strip on to the dorsal bulbar conjunctiva. *Never touch the cornea directly.*

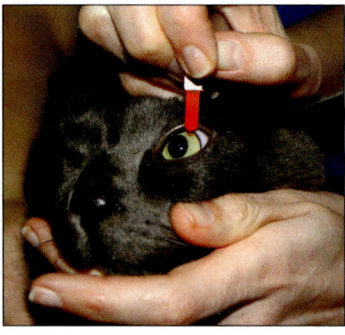

3 Irrigate the eye with further saline to flush excess fluorescein from the ocular surface. This avoids false negative and possible epitheliotoxic effects.

4 Examine the eye using a blue light source. Positive staining indicates a defect in the epithelium and, hence, an ulcer.

Orthopaedic examination

Indications/Use

- Lameness
- Abnormal gait
- Non-ambulatory
- Pyrexia of unknown origin

Observation

Take note of the following:

- Difficulty and/or reluctance in getting up or walking
- Failure to bear full weight on one or more limbs
- Shifting weight from one leg to the next while standing or sitting
- Posture
- Body shape abnormalities:
    - Focal muscle loss
    - Medial/lateral deviation of distal limbs
    - Limb hyperflexion or hyperextension
    - Angular or rotational deformities
- Evidence of old injuries; in particular, check feet, nails, pads and interdigital skin

Gait examination

- The animal should be observed walking and at moderate pace, both toward and away from the veterinary surgeon, on a firm level surface, as well as in front of or around the veterinary surgeon:
    - For most dogs this is best accomplished outdoors with the animal on a lead
    - Cats and very small dogs are best observed walking around the consulting room
    - Assessment walking up and down stairs can be helpful in some circumstances.
- Assess for:
    - Thoracic limb lameness:
        - A downward nod of the head as the 'sound' limb is placed to the ground
        - Lifting of the head as the lame limb strikes the ground
    - Pelvic limb lameness:
        - 'Hiking up' of the gluteal region on the lame side during weight bearing
        - 'Bunny hopping' gait in bilaterally affected animals
    - Swinging leg lameness:
        - Seen while the affected limb is in flight
        - Characteristic pattern of movement, depending upon the injury. For example:
            - Pelvic limb: contracture of the gracilis muscle results in outward rotation of the tarsus, with inward rotation of the foot

- – Thoracic limb: contracture of infraspinatus will cause the foot to swing in a lateral arc during protraction
- A shortened gait or reluctance to move a joint or joints through the full range of motion
- Abnormal flicking forward of the feet during protraction, e.g. due to reluctance to flex the elbows
- Neurological problems leading to paresis (weakness), ataxia (incoordination), spasticity (stiffness) or hypermetria. *These should be distinguished from lameness due to orthopaedic disorders by performing a full **neurological examination**.*

Palpation

- Palpation of the axial and appendicular skeleton should follow a set sequence:

  i. Palpate the spine, starting at the head and finishing at the tail
  ii. Palpate each limb from top to toe, comparing each leg with its opposite.

- Take note of the following:
  - Changes in muscles: check for asymmetries of shape due to swelling, atrophy, spasm, contracture or weakness
  - Anatomical deformities: check the spatial relationship of normal anatomical structures, particularly bony prominences. For example, craniodorsal hip luxation results in dorsal displacement of the greater trochanter and increased distance between the greater trochanter and ischiatic tuberosity
  - Swellings (may involve bones, joints or soft tissues)
  - Joint effusions: best appreciated where the joint capsule is least supported by the periarticular structures:
    - – Elbow effusions – caudolateral aspect
    - – Carpal effusions – dorsal aspect
    - – Interphalangeal effusions – dorsal aspect
    - – Stifle effusions – either side of the patellar ligament
    - – Tarsal effusions – just in front of the calcaneus.
  - Joint thickening
  - Pain from bone, muscle, tendons, neural tissue or joints.

Manipulation

- Manipulation of the axial and appendicular skeleton should follow a routine sequence:

  i. Flex the lower cervical spine and extend it in the axial plane and to the left and right
  ii. Flex, extend and rotate the lumbar spine
  iii. Manipulate each limb proximally to distally.

- Assess for:
  - Anatomical deformity or displacement (e.g. luxation, subluxation)

- Pain
- Range of movement of entire limb and each joint
- Crepitus
- The integrity of the supporting structures of each joint (collateral, dorsal, palmar, plantar ligaments, plus specialized structures such as cruciate ligaments and patella).

Shoulder

- Combined shoulder flexion and elbow extension, whilst placing direct pressure on the biceps tendon within the intertubercular groove, can identify bicipital tendon pain. To assess for medial instability the animal is placed in lateral recumbency and the thoracic limb is extended and maintained perpendicular to the spine. The forelimb is then adducted, whilst applying firm downward pressure over the acromion process. An increase in the angle of abduction compared to the contralateral limb is suggestive of medial instability.

Elbow

- Medial compartment pain can be detected by simultaneous flexion of the elbow and supination of the distal limb.

Carpus

- Extension is normally limited at 10 degrees of hyperextension.

Hip

- 110 degrees is the normal range of flexion and extension in a dog. (See also **Ortolani test**, below.)

Stifle

- Stability of the patella should be assessed in full extension and mild flexion to detect medial and lateral luxation, respectively. (See also **Cranial draw test** and **Tibial compression test**, below.)

Tarsus

- Collateral stability should be checked in both flexion and extension.
    - To assess the tibiotarsal joint, the base of the metatarsals should be grasped in one hand, whilst the lateral and medial malleoli are stabilized with the other.
    - To assess the tarsometatarsal and calcaneoquartal joints, the base of the metatarsals should be grasped in one hand, whilst the calcaneus is stabilized with the other.

Examination of the anaesthetized or sedated animal

- Once a seat of lameness has been identified in the conscious animal, additional information may be obtained under sedation or anaesthesia:
    - Some manipulations may be uncomfortable whether or not structures are abnormal (e.g. **Ortolani test**)

- A joint may be too painful to allow full assessment (**cranial draw test**, **tibial compression test**)
- Muscle tension in the conscious dog may mask instability
- Instability may be subtle.

Cranial draw test

Indications/Use

- To diagnose partial or complete rupture of the cranial cruciate ligament (CCL)
- **NB** This test does *not* identify isolated rupture of the caudolateral band of the CCL
- Often used in association with the **tibial compression test** (see below)

Contraindications

- Periarticular fibrosis and meniscal injury, with the caudal horn of the medial meniscus wedged between the femoral condyle and tibial plateau, may prevent cranial draw in a CCL-deficient stifle

Patient preparation and positioning

- Can be performed in the conscious animal. However, if the patient is tense (due to pain or temperament) or if the CCL is only partially torn, sedation or general anaesthesia may be required.
- A conscious patient may be restrained in a standing position on three legs, with the affected limb held off the ground.
- Sedated or anaesthetized patients may be positioned in lateral recumbency, with the affected limb uppermost.

Technique

1 Grasp the distal femur in one hand, placing the thumb over the lateral fabella and the index finger on the patella.
2 Use the other hand to grasp the proximal tibia, placing the thumb over the head of the fibula and the index finger on the tibial crest.
3 Apply a cranial force to the tibia while the stifle joint is held in full extension, and then while the joint is held in 30–60 degrees of flexion.

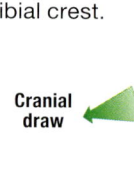

Cranial draw

Results

- Complete rupture of the CCL is associated with cranial displacement of the tibia relative to the femur, in both *extension and flexion*.
- Isolated rupture of the *craniomedial* band of the CCL is associated with cranial displacement of the tibia relative to the femur, in *flexion* only.
- A short cranial draw motion, with a distinct end point, may be detected in young animals and is normal.

Tibial compression test

Indications/Use

- To diagnose partial or complete rupture of the cranial cruciate ligament (CCL)
- **NB** Not all dogs with CCL disease have femorotibial instability that can be detected by this test
- Often used in association with the **cranial draw test** (see above)

Patient preparation and positioning

- Can be performed in the conscious animal. However, if the patient is tense (due to pain or temperament) or if the CCL is only partially torn, sedation or general anaesthesia is required.
- A conscious patient should be restrained in a standing position on three legs, with the affected limb held off the ground.
- Sedated or anaesthetized patients may be positioned in lateral recumbency, with the affected limb uppermost.

Technique

1 Grasp and maintain the distal femur in a fixed position with one hand, placing the thumb over the lateral fabella and the index finger lightly on the tibial crest.
2 Use the other hand to grasp the metatarsal region.
3 Maintain the stifle joint in slight flexion, while slowly flexing the hock.

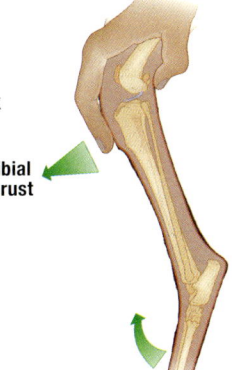

Tibial thrust

Results

- Cranial displacement (tibial thrust) of the tibial crest relative to the femur is suggestive of CCL injury.

Ortolani test

Indications/Use

- To detect hip laxity in the young dog (to support a diagnosis of hip dysplasia)

> **NOTE**
>
> Not all dogs with hip dysplasia show a positive Ortolani sign. For example, dogs with gross subluxation or luxation of the femoral head, and dogs in which capsular fibrosis has stabilized the hip joint will not show the sign.

Patient preparation and positioning

- May be attempted in the conscious animal but is potentially painful and therefore best performed with the dog heavily sedated or under general anaesthesia.
- The animal may be positioned in lateral or dorsal recumbency. The description below applies to lateral recumbency.

Technique

1 Position the stifle in mild flexion and grasp it with one hand, with the other hand placed on the dorsal aspect of the pelvis to stabilize it.

2 Apply firm pressure to the stifle in a dorsal direction in an attempt to subluxate the hip joint.

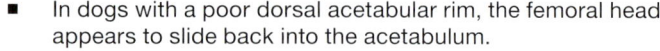

'Click'

3 Whilst maintaining dorsal pressure on the stifle, gently abduct the limb until a 'click' or 'clunk' is detected.

   ■ If the dorsal acetabular rim is intact, the femoral head falls abruptly into the acetabulum.

   ■ In dogs with a poor dorsal acetabular rim, the femoral head appears to slide back into the acetabulum.

4 Whilst maintaining dorsal pressure on the stifle, if the limb is now adducted, re-luxation of the hip will occur.

Results

■ The 'click' or 'clunk' (see Step 3) represents the relocation of the femoral head within the acetabulum. This is the positive Ortolani sign, consistent with hip joint laxity.

Assessment of the nervous system

■ An orthopaedic examination should *routinely* include assessment of deep and superficial pain perception, proprioception in all four limbs, and spinal reflexes in the limbs (see **Neurological examination**).

A

Abdominocentesis

Indications/Use

- To obtain abdominal fluid for analysis in cases of abdominal effusion (diagnostic abdominocentesis)
- To remove abdominal fluid in animals that have clinical signs associated with a large volume of fluid, e.g. respiratory distress due to the pressure on the diaphragm (therapeutic abdominocentesis)

Contraindications

- Coagulopathy
- Marked distension of an abdominal viscus
- Marked organomegaly

Equipment

- As required for **Aseptic preparation – (a) non-surgical procedures**
- **For diagnostic abdominocentesis:**
  - Hypodermic needles:
    - Dogs: 21 G; 1 to 1.5 inch
    - Cats: 23 G; ¾ inch
  - 5 ml syringe
- **For therapeutic abdominocentesis:**
  - 21 G 1 inch butterfly catheter attached to a 3-way tap
  - 20 ml syringe
- EDTA, plain and sterile collection tubes
- Microscope slides

Patient preparation and positioning

- Depending on the temperament of the patient, sedation may be required.
- The patient should be restrained in lateral recumbency, with its feet towards the clinician.
- It may be necessary to empty the patient's bladder by manual expression or **urethral catheterization** to reduce the risk of accidental cystocentesis.
- **Aseptic preparation – (a) non-surgical procedures** is carried out on an area approximately 10 cm x 10 cm, centred on the umbilicus, and a fenestrated drape placed.

Technique

- Diagnostic abdominocentesis is performed using either a single-site centesis or a four-quadrant approach. In patients with smaller effusions, the chances of fluid retrieval can also be increased by using ultrasound guidance.
- Therapeutic abdominocentesis is performed using a single-site centesis.
- For single-site centesis, the needle or butterfly catheter is inserted at right angles to the skin, 1–2 cm caudal to the umbilicus and 1 cm beneath the midline.

- For centesis using the four-quadrant approach, approximate needle insertion sites are indicated in the figure.

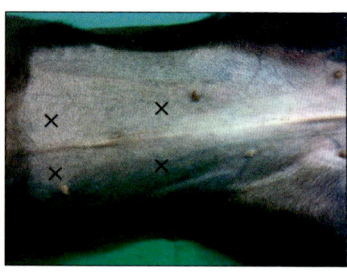

Black crosses indicate approximate sites, with the umbilicus central; the head is to the left

1 Insert the needle through the skin and abdominal wall, and twist it slightly to encourage fluid flow.

   i The needle should be inserted without a syringe attached. An open needle is more likely to result in fluid flow, as suction with a syringe will draw the omentum or viscera on to the needle.

   ii If using a butterfly catheter, this can be connected to a 3-way tap and syringe as it is inserted.

2 If using a needle, allow fluid to drip into a sampling tube.

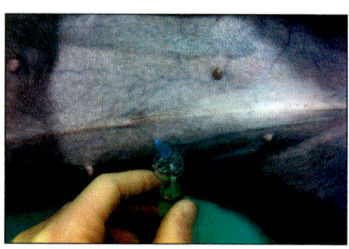

3 If no fluid is obtained, apply slight negative pressure with a 5 ml syringe.

4 If fluid is still not obtained, the needle can be reinserted in different locations using the four-quadrant approach (see above).

5 If there is still a suspicion of abdominal fluid, **diagnostic peritoneal lavage** can be performed.

Sample handling

- Place fluid in an EDTA tube for total nucleated cell count and cytology.
- Place fluid in a plain tube for total protein and any other biochemical or serological tests.
- A sample in a sterile plain tube can be submitted for bacteriological culture if necessary.
- Make several fresh air-dried smears (unstained).

Potential complications

- If blood is aspirated: stop the aspiration, place the blood in a glass tube and observe for clot formation. Blood from the abdominal cavity, i.e. haemorrhagic effusions, will not clot, whereas blood from a vessel or organ *will* clot.

If bleeding persists, abdominal pressure should be applied by way of manual compression or a pressure bandage
- Puncture of the GI tract: if fluid suggestive of GI contents is obtained, indicating that the GI tract has been punctured, any hole should seal when the needle is removed. The patient should, however, be monitored for developing peritonitis
- Continued drainage after needle removal: in some animals with large abdominal effusions, the centesis hole may continue to drain fluid. If this occurs, a pressure dressing may be applied

---

FURTHER INFORMATION

For interpretation of the results of fluid analysis, see the *BSAVA Manual of Canine and Feline Clinical Pathology*.

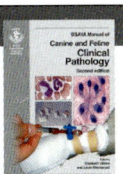

ACTH response test

Indications/Use
- Aid to the diagnosis of canine hyperadrenocorticism (HAC). Identifies >50% of dogs with adrenal-dependent HAC and about 85% of dogs with pituitary-dependent HAC
- Aid to the diagnosis of feline hyperadrenocorticism. Identifies approximately 50% of cases
- Monitoring trilostane or mitotane therapy
- Diagnosis of hypoadrenocorticism

Equipment
- As for **Blood sampling – (b) venous**
- Synthetic ACTH (0.25 mg/ml solution) (Tetracosactide, Tetracosactrin)
- Hypodermic needles: 21 G; ¾ to 1 inch
- Intravenous catheter
- 1 ml syringe
- Heparin or plain tubes: blood samples for cortisol measurements can be collected into heparin or plain tubes

Patient preparation and positioning
- The patient should be conscious.
- The patient is restrained in sternal recumbency or in a sitting position for collection of blood from the jugular vein, and then for intravenous injection into the cephalic vein (see **Blood sampling – (b) venous**).
- The area over the vessel to be sampled is clipped.
- Using cotton wool or soft swabs, the clipped area is wiped with 4% chlorhexidine gluconate or 10% povidone–iodine followed by 70% surgical spirit.

A

Technique

1 Collect a blood sample (approximately 2 ml) *from the jugular vein* (see **Blood sampling – (b) venous**) for basal cortisol concentration.
2 Inject 0.25 mg of synthetic ACTH *into the cephalic vein*. **NB In dogs <5 kg and cats, use only 0.125 mg**.

> **PRACTICAL TIP**
>
> When dealing with a very small dose of synthetic ACTH, it is preferable to place an **intravenous catheter** to ensure that the entire dose is administered.

3 Collect post-ACTH blood sample(s) (approximately 2 ml) *from the jugular vein* and place into separate heparin or plain tubes, at:
- 60 minutes (dogs)
- 60 and 90 minutes (cats).
4 Ensure the tubes are labelled correctly.
5 Separate the serum (plain tubes) and plasma (heparin tubes) samples prior to sending to the laboratory.

> **FURTHER INFORMATION**
>
> For interpretation of the ACTH response test results, see the *BSAVA Manual of Canine and Feline Endocrinology*.

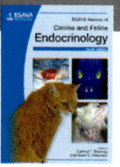

Anaphylaxis – emergency treatment

Identification

Anaphylaxis is an acute severe allergic reaction characterized by venous and arteriolar dilation and increased capillary permeability, which, in severe cases, result in decreased venous return to the heart, hypotension and hypoperfusion. Signs of anaphylaxis include:

- Angioedema: this commonly results in swelling of the face and distal limbs, but can include swelling of the pharynx and larynx.
- Bronchospasm
- Pruritus
- Urticaria: raised red skin wheals or hives
- Vomiting
- Anaphylactic shock

Procedure

1 Perform a rapid assessment of the airway, respiration and circulation.

2 If upper airway obstruction is evident with spontaneous respiration:
- Perform endotracheal (ET) intubation with sedation as required
- Administer supplemental oxygen as required: if measurements of oxygen are unavailable administer 100% oxygen.

3 Establish vascular access.

4 In life-threatening cases with evidence of upper airway obstruction or cardiovascular collapse (hypotension, bradycardia), give 0.02 mg/kg adrenaline i.v. slowly. *(Adrenaline can be given into the trachea if intravenous access is difficult, but may be ineffective. Insert a dog urinary catheter via the ET tube to the level of the carina. Dilute adrenaline with saline or sterile water.)*

- Initiate monitoring of ECG, S_pO_2, $ETCO_2$, blood pressure, venous blood gas, acid–base and electrolyte status.
- Monitor for adrenaline-induced arrhythmias and hypertension.

5 Treat hypoperfusion with intravenous fluid therapy and vasopressors as required.
- Crystalloids should be administered in boluses, as required, to achieve normotension (mean arterial pressure of 80–120 mmHg, systolic arterial pressure of 100–200 mmHg) and good perfusion (lactate <2.5 mmol/l).
- Vasopressors, such as dobutamine (5–15 µg/kg/min) or dopamine (3–10 µg/kg/min), should be considered if hypotension is unresponsive to fluid therapy.

6 Following initial emergency treatment, if bronchospasm and angioedema persist, consider dexamethasone (0.5 mg/kg i.v. once).

7 Long-term prophylaxis requires identification and avoidance of the causative agent.

FURTHER INFORMATION

For further discussion of the treatment of hypovolaemic shock see the *BSAVA Manual of Canine and Feline Emergency and Critical Care.*

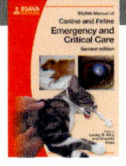

Arthrocentesis

Indications/Use

- Joint disease of unknown aetiology
- Pain on manipulation of a joint
- Joint effusion
- Joint heat

A
B
C
D
E
F
G
H
I
J
K
L
M
N
O
P
Q
R
S
T
U
V
W
X
Y
Z

- Periarticular thickening
- Suspected immune-mediated joint disease (e.g. pyrexia of unknown origin)
- Suspected infective arthritis
- Monitoring response to therapy in infective arthritis and immune-mediated polyarthritis

Contraindications

- Severe coagulopathy

Equipment

- As required for **Aseptic preparation – (a) non-surgical procedures**

> ### GLOVES
> Sterile gloves should be worn if the clinician wishes to palpate bony landmarks and the needle insertion site. As experience is gained, such palpation is not necessary and gloves may not be required, provided the needle insertion point is not touched.

- Hypodermic needles: 21–23 G; $5/8$ to 1.5 inch, depending on joint size
- 2–10 ml syringes (Larger syringe sizes allow better negative pressure, especially if joint fluid is expected to be of normal viscosity. A 10 ml syringe can be used if there is a palpable effusion and large amounts of fluid are expected)
- Microscope slides
- EDTA and heparin collection tubes
- Blood culture bottle/bacteriology swab in transport medium

Patient preparation and positioning

- Heavy sedation or general anaesthesia is required.
- The patient is placed in lateral recumbency, with the affected joint uppermost.
- The joint for aspiration will often be dictated by the findings on clinical examination, e.g. pain on joint manipulation, palpable effusion.
- An assistant may be required to hold the limb and flex or extend the joint as required.
- **Aseptic preparation – (a) non-surgical procedures** is performed on an area approximately 5 cm x 5 cm over the site for arthrocentesis.

Technique

1. **a. Carpus:** The antebrachiocarpal (radiocarpal) joint is generally the most accessible. With the carpus partially to fully flexed, the antebrachiocarpal joint is palpable as a depression just distal to the radius. Insert the needle

medial to the common digital extensor tendon and cephalic vein, which pass over the centre of the joint space. The needle insertion site is just lateral to the tendon of extensor carpi radialis. The antebrachiocarpal joint does not communicate with the other carpal joints. If no fluid is obtained, or blood contamination occurs, try tapping the intercarpal joint to obtain a sample. The intercarpal and carpometacarpal joints communicate.

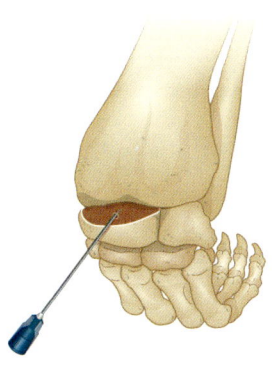 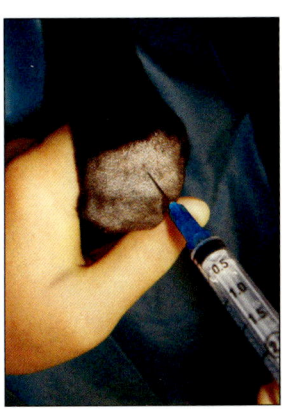

b. **Tarsus (hock):** The talocrural joint space is most readily aspirated. Flex and extend the talocrural joint to locate the position of the joint. With the joint in a neutral position, insert the needle on the dorsolateral aspect of the talocrural joint, just medial to the palpable lateral malleolus of the fibula, and advance it towards the plantaromedial aspect of the joint. *Alternative:* The plantarolateral joint space may be aspirated by inserting the needle parallel to the calcaneus, just medial to the lateral malleolus.

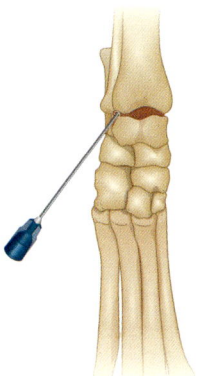 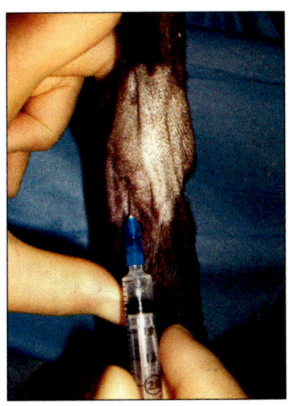

A

c. **Stifle:** The joint capsule of the stifle has three sacs, all of which communicate. With the joint partially flexed, apply digital pressure to the joint capsule on the medial side of the patellar ligament. Introduce the needle just lateral to the straight patellar ligament, midway between the femur and tibia. Direct the needle into the joint space, through the fat pad, towards the intercondylar space in the centre of the joint. If no synovial fluid is aspirated, the needle should be moved inwards or outwards and re-aspiration attempted, as the needle tip may be located in the fat pad.

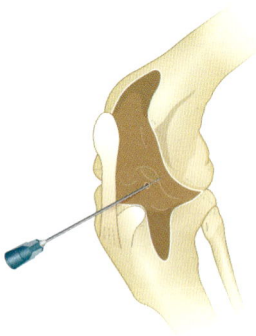
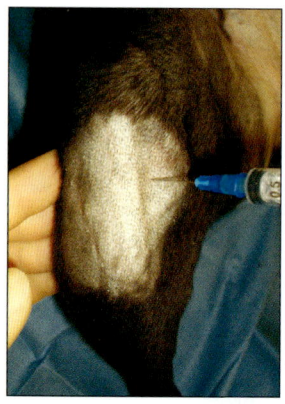

Alternative: The needle can be inserted parallel to the straight patellar ligament, midway between the tibial tuberosity and patella. The tip of the needle is directed lateral to the patella in the lateral parapatellar joint pouch.

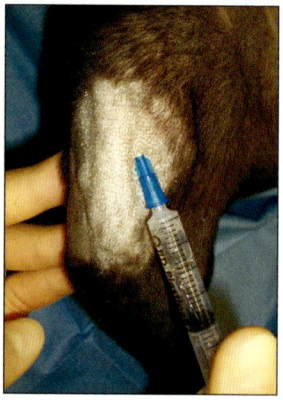

d. **Elbow:** The caudolateral approach is the easiest and most atraumatic. Flex the elbow to approximately 45 degrees, and palpate the lateral condyle of the humerus and the olecranon. Advance the needle parallel to the long axis of the ulna, midway between these two landmarks. The needle should slide between the lateral epicondylar crest of the humerus and the anconeal process of the ulna. Once the needle is through the skin, it is usually necessary to apply slight downward (medial) pressure on the shaft of the needle with the thumb while it is advanced towards the joint space. This is necessary in order to maintain the needle's caudal-to-cranial orientation parallel to the olecranon and straight into the joint. In most cases the needle needs to be inserted deep into the joint before fluid is aspirated.

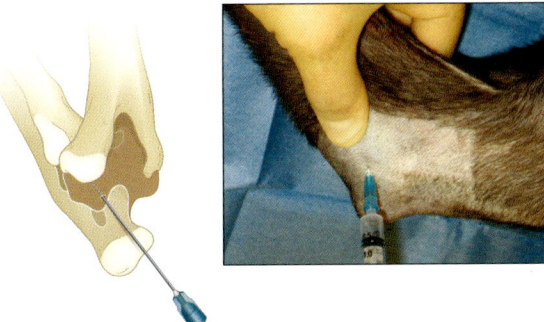

e. **Shoulder:** With the dog in lateral recumbency, hold the shoulder in partial flexion and maintain the limb parallel to the table as if the animal were standing and weightbearing. Palpate the acromion process and introduce the needle perpendicular to the skin directly distal to the acromion. Distal traction can be applied to the limb by an assistant to open the joint space if required. If the needle hits bone, gently 'walk' the needle a few millimetres proximally or distally until the joint is penetrated.

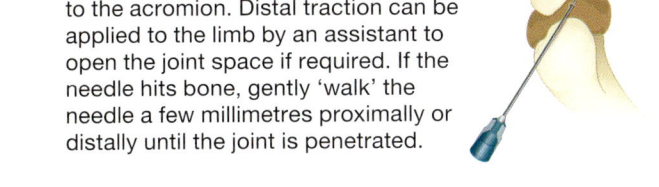

2 Attach a syringe to the needle and gently aspirate until synovial fluid appears in the hub of the needle.

3 Once sufficient fluid has entered the syringe (which may only be a hubful), release the suction to minimize inadvertent aspiration of blood, before withdrawing the needle and syringe. To reduce the chance of blood contamination further, the syringe can be removed from the needle prior to needle removal from the joint space.

Sample handling

■ To maximize preservation of cell morphology, smears should be made immediately and allowed to air dry. The squash technique should be used – see **Fine needle aspiration**.

■ If more than approximately 0.2–0.3 ml of fluid is obtained, this can be placed in an EDTA tube for cytological evaluation and total nucleated cell count.

A

- Heparin is the preferred anticoagulant for the mucin precipitation test and for measurement of viscosity; however, these tests are rarely performed in clinical practice.
- If bacterial infective arthritis is suspected, synovial fluid should be placed in blood culture media. Alternatively, a few drops of fluid can be placed on a sterile bacteriology swab placed in a commercial transport medium (e.g. Amies charcoal).

Potential complications

- Iatrogenic articular cartilage damage
- Joint infection
- Haemorrhage

> **FURTHER INFORMATION**
>
> Details of the evaluation of synovial fluid are given in the *BSAVA Manual of Canine and Feline Clinical Pathology* and in the *BSAVA Manual of Canine and Feline Musculoskeletal Disorders*.

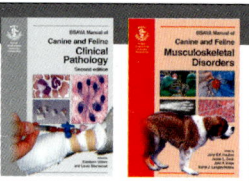

Aseptic preparation – (a) non-surgical procedures

Indications/Use

- Skin preparation for any veterinary procedure requiring aseptic technique, where there is a risk of iatrogenic contamination leading to infection

Equipment

- Regularly maintained clean, sharp electric clippers
- Vacuum cleaner
- Cotton wool or soft swabs
- Container to hold used cotton wool or soft swabs
- Tap water
- Appropriate antiseptic
    - For routine preparation of healthy skin, 4% chlorhexidine gluconate or 10% povidone–iodine, used in combination with 70% surgical spirit, is appropriate
    - Chlorhexidine gluconate or povidone–iodine should be avoided in animals with known skin sensitivities to either of these antiseptics
    - Chlorhexidine gluconate is specifically toxic to the conjunctiva, cornea, meninges and middle and inner ear: 0.2% povidone–iodine solution without alcohol is recommended for preparation of the periocular area but

must *not* be allowed to contact the cornea; 1% povidone–iodine solution without alcohol is recommended for preparation of the external ear canal for surgery

- Alcohol has a desiccating effect when applied to mucous membranes and should *not* be used for surgeries close to, or involving, mucous membranes (e.g. intraoral surgery)

> **NOTE**
>
> Sterile applicators containing 2% chlorhexidine gluconate and 70% isopropyl alcohol, designed specifically for skin antisepsis are now available. They should be used according to the manufacturer's recommendations, rather than following the technique below.

- The application of antiseptics directly to open wounds is not recommended
- Appropriate sterile skin drapes; these may be:
  - Well maintained and laundered cloth drapes
  - Disposable semi-impermeable synthetic drapes
  - Or one sterile fenestrated drape may be appropriate for non-surgical procedures

Technique

1 Hair removal
  - Remove hair from the procedure site with electric clippers.
  - Include margins up to 15 cm around the proposed procedural site. Clip sufficient hair to avoid contamination of the veterinary surgeon, the procedural site and sterile equipment.
  - Remove clipped hair from the procedural site. A vacuum cleaner may be used with anaesthetized animals, but using a vacuum cleaner around a conscious or sedated animal may cause undue distress to the patient.

2 Skin preparation
  - Apply antiseptic of an appropriate concentration to balls of damp cotton wool or swabs.
  - Clean the clipped area by applying gentle pressure in a circular motion, beginning at the proposed procedural site (e.g. site of needle insertion) and working outwards in concentric circles. Use a fresh cotton wool ball or swab each time cleaning is returned to the centre of the procedural site.
  - Continue cleaning for at least 3 minutes until no dirt can be seen grossly on the cotton wool balls or swabs.
  - Dampen the hair around the clipped area to flatten it away from the procedural site.
  - Squirt or gently spray surgical spirit on to the procedural site. **NB Do NOT use surgical spirit to prepare sites that include the eyes or mucous membranes.**

A

3 Draping
- Draping may not be required for short minor procedures where the risk of contamination of the procedural site and sterile equipment is negligible (e.g. fine needle aspiration of skin masses, arthrocentesis).
- **Draping should always be used if in doubt.** A simple fenestrated drape laid over the site may be sufficient to prevent contamination of a procedural site. For short procedures and procedures performed in non-anaesthetized patients, towel clamps are, respectively, not required and not advised.

> **NOTE**
>
> Draping should be performed by a veterinary surgeon or nurse who has scrubbed hands and is wearing sterile gloves.

Potential complications

- Clipper rash
- Dermatitis due to idiosyncratic reaction to antiseptic
- Break in asepsis

Aseptic preparation – (b) surgical procedures

Indications/Use

- Skin preparation for all surgical procedures

Equipment

- Regularly maintained clean, sharp electric clippers
- Vacuum cleaner
- Cotton wool or soft swabs
- Container to hold used cotton wool or soft swabs
- Tap water
- Appropriate antiseptic
  - For routine preparation of healthy skin, 4% chlorhexidine gluconate or 10% povidone–iodine, used in combination with 70% surgical spirit, is appropriate
  - Chlorhexidine gluconate or povidone–iodine should be avoided in animals with known skin sensitivities to either of these antiseptics
  - Chlorhexidine gluconate is specifically toxic to the conjunctiva, cornea, meninges and middle and inner ear; 0.2% povidone–iodine solution without alcohol is recommended for preparation of the periocular area but must *not* be allowed to contact the cornea; 1% povidone–

iodine solution without alcohol is recommended for preparation of the external ear canal for surgery
- Alcohol has a desiccating effect when applied to mucous membranes and should *not* be used for surgeries close to, or involving, mucous membranes (e.g. intraoral surgery)

> **NOTE**
>
> Sterile applicators containing 2% chlorhexidine gluconate and 70% isopropyl alcohol, designed specifically for skin antisepsis are now available. They should be used according to the manufacturer's recommendations, rather than following the technique below, and can be used for the final skin preparation in the operating theatre.

- The application of antiseptics directly to open wounds is not recommended
- Appropriate sterile skin drapes: these may be well maintained and laundered cloth drapes, or disposable semi-impermeable synthetic drapes
  - 4 sterile field drapes are appropriate for most surgical operations
  - Sterile transparent adherent plastic drapes and sterile skin towels may be used at the veterinary surgeon's discretion
- Sterile towel clamps

Technique

1 Hair removal
   - Remove hair from the surgical site with electric clippers.
   - Include margins of at least 15 cm around the proposed surgical incision.
   - Remove clipped hair immediately with a vacuum cleaner.
   - For operations on limbs, clip the entire limb apart from the phalanges. Phalanges should only be clipped when they are included in the surgical field. Wrap the unclipped phalanges and as much of the paw as the surgical site permits in a semi-impermeable, self-adhesive, non-adherent outer bandage material.

2 Skin preparation outside the operating room
   - Apply antiseptic of an appropriate concentration to balls of damp cotton wool or soft cotton swabs.
   - Clean the clipped area by applying gentle pressure in a circular motion, beginning at the proposed incision site and working outwards in concentric circles. Use a fresh cotton wool ball or swab each time cleaning is returned to the incision site.
   - Continue cleaning until no dirt can be seen grossly on the cotton wool balls or swabs.
   - For operations including the phalanges, soak the paw in a dilute solution of antiseptic for 3 minutes or until all gross

A

dirt has been removed.
- Dampen the hair around the clipped area to flatten it away from the surgical site.

3 Patient transfer to the operating room
- Transfer the patient to the operating room.
- Position the patient appropriately for surgery, using sandbags and ties.
- For limb operations, the limb is hung from the toes or paw. This is carried out using ropes tied to vertical stands, with top horizontal crossbars that can be raised and lowered.

4 Skin preparation inside the operating room
- Apply antiseptic of an appropriate concentration to balls of damp cotton wool or swabs.
- Clean the clipped area by applying gentle pressure in a circular motion beginning at the proposed incision site and working outwards in concentric circles. Use a fresh cotton wool ball or swab each time cleaning is returned to the incision site.
- Continue this scrubbing for at least 3 minutes.
- Squirt or gently spray surgical spirit on to the surgical site. **NB Do NOT use surgical spirit to prepare surgical sites that include the eyes or mucous membranes.**

5 Draping
- Sterile surgical drapes are placed around the surgical field. Draping should leave exposed only the aseptically prepared skin and cover all hair. Drapes are secured in place with towel clamps placed at each of the four corners of the surgical field and then along the sides of the surgical field as necessary.
- Sterile surgical skin towels may be attached to the edges of the skin incision using towel clamps following the initial skin incision. Such skin draping has not been shown to decrease the incidence of surgical site infection, but is preferred by some surgeons.
- A sterile transparent adherent plastic drape may be used to cover skin that is exposed following routine draping. This may decrease the incidence of surgical site infection and is preferred by many surgeons, especially for orthopaedic procedures.
- For limb operations, a non-scrubbed assistant passes the foot to the surgeon. The surgeon covers the foot with an appropriately sized sterile surgical drape, which is wrapped around the distal limb and secured with a towel clamp. The surgeon avoids contacting the foot directly, so as to remain sterile. The entire distal limb including the towel clamp and drape are wrapped in a semi-impermeable, self-adhesive, non-adherent outer bandage material, which has been sterilized specifically for this purpose. The limb is then held by a sterile surgical assistant, while it is draped using four sterile surgical drapes as above.

NOTE

Draping should be performed by a veterinary surgeon or nurse who has scrubbed their lower arms and hands and is wearing a mask, hat, sterile gloves and gown.

Potential complications

- Clipper rash
- Dermatitis due to idiosyncratic reaction to antiseptic
- Break in asepsis

FURTHER INFORMATION

For more information on Aseptic technique, see the *BSAVA Manual of Canine and Feline Surgical Principles*.

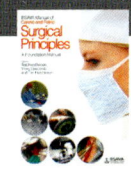

A
B
C
D
E
F
G
H
I
J
K
L
M
N
O
P
Q
R
S
T
U
V
W
X
Y
Z

Barium contrast media

There is a wide variety of preparations of barium sulphate used in veterinary radiography. None of these preparations is authorized for veterinary use and most are POM.

Formulation	Trade name	Comments
94% w/w granules to reconstitute as suspension	Baritop plus	200 g pack 1000 g pack
100% w/v suspension	Baritop 100	300 ml can
95% w/w vanilla-flavoured powder to reconstitute as a suspension	Barosperse	225 g bottle 900 g bottle
70% w/v raspberry flavoured paste	Intropaste	454 g tubes
95% w/w cherry flavoured powder to reconstitute as a suspension	Tonopaque	180 g bottle 1200 g bottle
98% w/w vanilla flavoured powder to reconstitute as a suspension	HD 200 plus	312 g bottle
100% w/v liquid barium suspension 105% w/v liquid barium suspension	Polibar	1900 ml
60% w/v liquid barium suspension	Liquid E-ZPaque	1900 ml
40% w/v liquid barium suspension	Varibar	
210% w/v liquid barium suspension	Maxibar	
98% w/v powder for suspension	E-Z-HD	
Barium-impregnated polyethylene spheres	BIPS	Large (5 mm diameter) and small (1.5 mm diameter) combined in capsules
Barium sulphate powder	Barium sulphate BP	500 g

Use

- Used for gastrointestinal (GI) contrast studies
- Barium sulphate has a higher atomic number than body tissues and therefore appears radiopaque. Barium sulphate is inert with no osmotic potential and is not absorbed or acted upon by alimentary secretions. Enables visualization of lumen of oesophagus and GI tract
- Barium-impregnated polyethylene spheres (BIPS) may be used to assess intestinal transit times and gastric emptying rate, and to detect obstructions
- As with all contrast studies, plain radiographs should be taken prior to administration of barium
- Barium paste is used for oesophageal studies as it adheres to mucosa. Barium can also be mixed with food to evaluate the

oesophagus, and may demonstrate strictures or dilatations not seen with liquid barium or paste
- Liquid barium may be used to evaluate any part of the GI tract and is used alone for evaluation of the stomach and intestines. Flavoured preparations designed for human use may be unpalatable for some animals. Mixing barium with methylcellulose may improve the quality of GI tract studies

Safety and handling

- Skin irritation may occur with skin contact.
- Take care not to spill barium on the patient's coat; clean off any spills carefully.

Contraindications and adverse reactions

- Barium is insoluble and should not be used outside the GI tract.
- If endoscopy is going to follow contrast radiography it is preferable to use a water-soluble contrast medium, as barium will prevent evaluation of the mucosa.
- Leakage of barium into body cavities may lead to granulomatous reactions or adhesions.
- If oesophageal or GI tract perforation is suspected, low-osmolar water-soluble contrast media should be used.
- Care should be employed when administering barium to dysphagic animals or those with severe oesophageal disease, as aspiration pneumonia may result.
- May cause constipation, transient diarrhoea and abdominal pain.

Barium studies of the gastrointestinal tract – (a) oesophagus

Indications/Use

- Regurgitation
- Retching
- Dysphagia
- Vomiting of undigested food soon after eating

ULTRASONOGRAPHY

Barium affects the ultrasonographic appearance of the GI tract. If ultrasonography is required, it should therefore be performed prior to the barium study.

WARNING

- Particular care should be taken when administering barium to animals with swallowing disorders, so as to minimize the risk of aspiration of contrast medium and subsequent inhalation pneumonia.

Contraindications

- Suspected or confirmed oesophageal perforation: use non-ionic **iodinated contrast media** instead

Equipment

- Barium sulphate (see **Barium contrast media**)
- Lukewarm water for dilution
- Soft tinned food
- Food bowl
- 20–60 ml syringe with catheter tip
- Radiographic or fluoroscopic equipment

> **OPTIONS**
>
> - Barium paste is primarily used to highlight abnormalities of oesophageal mucosa.
> - A barium meal (barium paste added to food) is best for identifying functional abnormalities.

Patient preparation and positioning

- The patient should be conscious if possible. Light sedation can be used if necessary, although this will increase the risk of contrast medium aspiration and may alter oesophageal function.
- Contrast medium should be administered orally, with the patient in a sitting or standing position.
- The animal is subsequently positioned for radiographs as detailed below.
- Alternatively, horizontal beam fluoroscopy can be performed with the patient in a standing position.

Technique

1 Take plain left lateral and dorsoventral radiographs of the thorax and cranial abdomen. This is important, as significant findings such as foreign material may be masked by contrast medium. These views also allow for the detection of any pre-existing aspiration pneumonia.

> **WARNING**
>
> - **If gross megaoesophagus is diagnosed on plain radiography, administration of barium is contraindicated because of the risk of aspiration pneumonia.**

2 Administer thick barium sulphate paste (60% w/v) orally, via a syringe at a dose of approximately 1 ml per 5 kg bodyweight. Barium paste will highlight mucosal abnormalities which could be obscured by the barium meal; whilst a barium meal will display gross structural abnormalities.

3 Immediately take either a right or left lateral radiograph of the cervical and thoracic oesophagus. Additional information may be

gained from a dorsoventral view, especially if a vascular ring anomaly is suspected.

4 If necessary, encourage the patient to eat a mixture of soft tinned food to which has been added approximately 20–30 ml of 100% w/v barium sulphate suspension, and repeat radiography.

Potential complications

- Aspiration pneumonia
- Vomiting
- Diarrhoea

Barium studies of the gastrointestinal tract – (b) stomach and small intestine

Indications/Use

- Persistent vomiting
- Haematemesis
- Displacement of the gastrointestinal (GI) tract associated with diaphragmatic rupture
- Assessment of GI tract displacement by changes in size or position of adjacent organs
- Unexplained dilatation of the small intestine

ULTRASONOGRAPHY

Barium affects the ultrasonographic appearance of the GI tract. If ultrasonography is required, it should therefore be performed prior to the barium study.

WARNING

- **Particular care should be taken when administering barium to animals with swallowing disorders, so as to minimize the risk of aspiration of contrast medium and subsequent inhalation pneumonia.**

Contraindications

- Suspected GI tract rupture
- Convincing evidence of small intestinal dilatation on plain films, with a strong suspicion of mechanical obstruction

Equipment

- Barium sulphate suspension (see **Barium contrast media**)
- Lukewarm water for dilution
- Soft tinned food
- Food bowl
- 20–60 ml syringe with catheter tip
- Radiographic equipment

B

Patient preparation and positioning

- For an elective examination, food should be withheld for 24 hours prior to the procedure.
- The patient should be conscious if possible. If sedation is necessary, acepromazine has been found to have the least effect on GI motility and will assist restraint and accurate positioning.
- Contrast medium should be administered orally, with the patient in a sitting or standing position.
- The animal is subsequently positioned for radiographs as detailed below.

Technique

1 Take plain lateral and ventrodorsal radiographs of the abdomen. This is important, as significant findings such as foreign material may be masked by contrast medium.
2 Administer approximately 10 ml/kg of barium sulphate suspension (30% w/v) orally via a syringe.
3 For a full evaluation of the stomach, take four views immediately following administration of the contrast medium: right lateral; left lateral; ventrodorsal; and dorsoventral. In each case the radiograph should be centred over the cranial abdomen at the level of the last rib.
4 To assess gastric emptying: take repeat radiographs of the stomach 5–10 minutes after the initial films to verify the presence of any observed lesions, and to assess normal onset of gastric emptying. Further films at 10–15 minute intervals may be required in cases of delayed gastric emptying.
5 To evaluate the small intestine: following the gastric examination, take lateral and ventrodorsal views at regular intervals, depending on the rate of passage in the individual case, until either a diagnosis has been reached or the barium has entered the large intestine. A film taken 24 hours after administration of the contrast medium should be used to demonstrate that all the contrast medium has reached the large intestine.

> **NOTE**
>
> If the barium study is performed to demonstrate displacement of the GI tract during the investigation of an abdominal mass or diaphragmatic rupture, it is more economical to omit the initial films and take radiographs 30–45 minutes after administration of contrast medium. By this time, the stomach and most of the small intestine should contain contrast medium.

Potential complications

- Aspiration pneumonia
- Vomiting
- Diarrhoea

Barium studies of the gastrointestinal tract – (c) large intestine

Indications/Use

- Tenesmus
- Melaena
- Chronic diarrhoea
- Identification of the position of the large intestine in relation to caudal abdominal/intrapelvic masses

---

ULTRASONOGRAPHY

Barium affects the ultrasonographic appearance of the GI tract. If ultrasonography is required, it should therefore be performed prior to the barium study.

Contraindications

- Large rectal or colonic mass that would preclude the passage of the tube for administering barium sulphate
- Suspected rupture of the lower GI tract

Equipment

- Barium sulphate suspension (see Barium contrast media)
- Equipment for giving an enema and administering contrast medium: 20–60 ml syringe; lukewarm water or saline; enema pump or tubing and funnel; lubricating gel such as K-Y jelly
- Radiographic equipment
- Foley catheter
- Suture material

Patient preparation and positioning

- For an elective examination, food should be withheld for 24 hours prior to the procedure.
- A rectal examination is required to ensure that it is safe to insert the enema and barium sulphate.
- At least one non-irritant cleansing enema (e.g. warm water) should be given 2–3 hours prior to the procedure, to evacuate the large intestine. This can be performed with the patient in lateral recumbency or standing and is usually best performed outside.
- The patient should be heavily sedated or anaesthetized. This will not interfere with the results of the contrast study.

Technique

1 Take plain lateral and ventrodorsal radiographs of the abdomen to assess patient preparation and whether further enemas are required.

B

2 Administer the diluted suspension of barium sulphate (20% w/v) slowly into the descending colon, using either an enema pump or a gravity-feed tube and funnel. The volume of contrast medium required is usually about 8 ml/kg bodyweight.

3 With a sedated or anaesthetized patient, leakage of contrast medium from the anus may occur. This can be prevented by administering the contrast medium via a Foley catheter, and securing the catheter within the rectum with a purse-string suture around the anus.

4 Take lateral and ventrodorsal radiographs of the abdomen as soon as the infusion of barium is complete.

5 A 'double contrast' study can also be performed, as this may allow better evaluation of mucosal detail. This is normally performed after the positive-contrast colonogram. As much barium as possible is drained out, followed by distending the colon with approximately 8 ml/kg of air. Lateral and ventrodorsal radiographs of the abdomen are then taken.

Potential complications

- Rupture of the lower GI tract
- Trauma to the lower GI tract
- Haematochezia
- Diarrhoea

Blood pressure measurement – (a) direct

Invasive blood pressure measurement by means of an arterial catheter is considered the 'gold standard' technique but is technically demanding in terms of placement of the catheter, maintaining patency of the arterial catheter and ensuring accurate 'zeroing' of the apparatus to ambient air at the level of the right atrium.

Indications/Use

- Monitoring arterial blood pressure in critically ill patients
- Monitoring arterial blood pressure during anaesthesia
- *Arterial catheters can also be used for serial collection of arterial blood samples for blood gas analysis in animals with pulmonary disease*

Contraindications

- Coagulopathy
- Arterial catheters should not be placed at sites where risk of bacterial contamination and infection are high, e.g. due to local tissue damage, local skin infection, diarrhoea, urinary incontinence

Equipment

- No. 11 scalpel
- 20–22 G peripheral venous over-the-needle catheter
- T-connector or extension set containing heparinized saline (1 IU of heparin per ml of 0.9% saline)
- 70% surgical spirit
- Adhesive tape
- Soft padded bandage and outer protective bandage
- Non-compliant manometer tubing
- Pressure transducer: must be 'zeroed' to ambient air at the level of the right atrium
- Display monitor
- Pressurized continuous flush system

Patient preparation and positioning

- The patient should be positioned in lateral recumbency.
- The patient's limb must be held still; this can be achieved by manual restraint.
- For monitoring of the anaesthetized patient, arterial catheters should be placed soon after anaesthetic induction, and before the animal's blood pressure falls, as low BP makes palpation of a peripheral arterial pulse more challenging.

Sites

- The dorsal pedal artery in the hindpaw is most commonly used.
- Other arteries that may be used include: the femoral artery; auricular artery; and palmar metacarpal artery in the forepaw.

Technique

1 Place a catheter into a peripheral artery.
   - Palpate the arterial pulse.
   - The skin overlying the artery is clipped, then sprayed or lightly wiped with surgical spirit. Excessive scrubbing/wiping of the skin should be avoided, as this may result in spasm of the artery.
   - Make a small stab incision in the skin overlying the arterial pulse.
   - A peripheral venous catheter is placed through the skin incision and then inserted into the artery using short, firm, purposeful movements to push the stylet and catheter through the muscular wall of the artery. For entry into the artery, the catheter should be positioned at a slight angle to the artery – approximately 10–30 degrees.
   - The dorsal pedal artery runs at about 30 degrees to the long axis of the metatarsus from medial to lateral. During

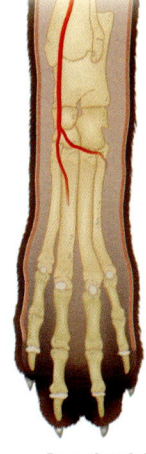

Dorsal pedal artery

catheter placement palpate the arterial pulse constantly, proximal to the site of entry of the catheter into the artery. This allows the operator to guide the catheter tip towards the artery, which cannot be seen.

- As soon as arterial blood is seen in the flash chamber of the catheter, the stylet and catheter are lowered to a position parallel to the artery and advanced together a little further into the artery, before the catheter is advanced over the stylet and completely into the artery.
- Withdraw the catheter stylet and attach a T-connector or extension set containing heparinized saline to the catheter. Arterial blood should be seen to pulsate within the hub of the catheter or T-connector.
- The catheter should be secured firmly in place with adhesive tape and covered with a bandage.

WARNING

- **The bandage over an arterial catheter must be labelled clearly to avoid inadvertent administration of fluids or drugs into an artery.**

---

2   Connect the T-connector to a pressure transducer via non-compliant tubing filled with heparinized saline.

3   To allow trouble-free continuous monitoring (avoiding clotting in the arterial line), the set-up is combined with a pressurized continuous flush system. If this is not available, arterial catheters should be flushed hourly.

4   The transducer–monitor combination gives a continuous reading of blood pressure and shows the pressure waveform. Systolic and diastolic pressures are taken as the cyclic maximum and minimum pressures, respectively. Mean pressure is calculated automatically. Arterial blood pressure monitoring is usually continuous.

5   On removal of the catheter, apply direct pressure to the artery for 5 minutes, then wrap with a light pressure dressing, e.g. folded gauze swab secured in place over the artery with adhesive tape.

Potential complications

- Excessive arterial bleeding/exsanguination following a failed attempt at catheterization or accidental removal of the catheter
- Vascular damage and subsequent tissue necrosis distal to the catheter. The risk of this complication can be minimized by:
  - Avoiding placing adhesive tape too tightly around the paw
  - Never using arterial catheters for giving drugs or fluids
  - Regular monitoring of the catheter and paw; arterial catheters should be checked every hour
  - Prompt removal of arterial catheters when they are no longer required

- Infection
- Thrombosis/thromboembolism
- Embolism of a piece of catheter due to accidental transection of the catheter with a blade or scissors
- Air embolism

Blood pressure measurement – (b) indirect

Non-invasive blood pressure measurements are technically less demanding than invasive measurements and can be rapidly applied in the emergency situation, although they might not fulfil the expectations of reliability and accuracy. There are two non-invasive methods in general use: the oscillometric method and the Doppler method. Both require a cuff.

Indications/Use

- To assess cardiovascular function
- Routine monitoring during anaesthesia

Equipment

- Doppler ultrasound probe
- Coupling gel
- Adhesive tape
- Inflatable cuff attached to a manometer
  OR
  Oscillometric blood pressure monitor with cuffs

> **CUFF SIZE**
>
> The proper cuff width is 40% of the circumference of the site where the cuff will be placed. Cuffs that are too wide lead to falsely low readings; those that are too narrow lead to falsely high readings.

Patient preparation and positioning

- Can be performed on conscious, sedated or anaesthetized animals.

> **NOTE**
>
> Assessment of general cardiovascular status should be made in the absence of sedative and anaesthetic drugs.

- For conscious animals, it is important that they are relaxed. A quiet, stress-free environment is ideal. Allow the animal a period of at least 5–10 minutes to relax.
- The limb used should not be weight-bearing and the animal should be positioned such that the cuff is at the level of the right atrium.

- For the Doppler technique it is necessary to prepare the skin overlying the artery to be used for blood pressure measurement. Normally the fur should be removed by shaving. However, in cats with short fur, wiping down the fur with surgical spirit may be adequate. Common sites for the detection of an arterial pulse using the Doppler technique are:
  - The palmar arterial arch, on the ventral aspect of the proximal metacarpal region
  - The plantar arterial arch, on the ventral aspect of the proximal metatarsal region
  - The median caudal artery on the ventral aspect of the tail.

Technique

Doppler ultrasound

An inflatable cuff attached to a manometer occludes an artery, and a piezoelectric crystal placed over the artery distal to the cuff detects flow. The re-entry of blood into the artery as the cuff is released causes a frequency change (Doppler shift) in the sound waves. This is detected by the piezoelectric crystal and converted to a sound that is detected by the operator. **This method primarily measures systolic pressure. Recordings of diastolic pressures may be inaccurate.**

1 Apply coupling gel directly to the transducer with the machine switched off.
2 Turn the machine on. Gently position the Doppler ultrasound probe over the prepared skin. Listen carefully for a pulse signal, moving the probe gently until a clear signal can be heard. Secure the probe to the prepared area with adhesive tape.
3 If no signal is heard, consider:
  i Applying more coupling gel
  ii Securing the probe to the prepared skin before hearing a signal. Excessive digital pressure on the probe may occlude the artery, whereas the pressure from the tape alone may be less, allowing the pulse signal to be heard.

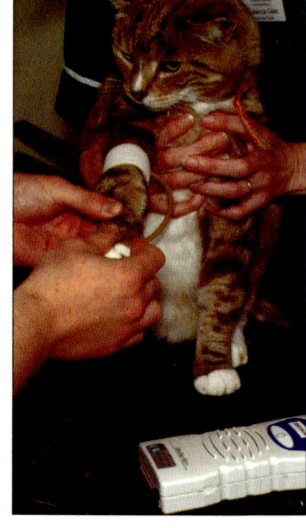

4 Attach the cuff to a handheld sphygmomanometer. Place the cuff around the limb or tail proximal to the probe, avoiding the joints. In dogs, the cuff should be applied snugly enough to allow insertion of only a small finger between the cuff and the leg or tail. Most cuffs have a mark that should be placed directly over the artery.

> **PRACTICAL TIP**
>
> If the cuff is applied too tightly, the measurement will be erroneously low because the cuff partly occludes the artery; if applied too loosely, the measurement will be erroneously high because excessive cuff pressure will be required to occlude the artery.

5 Gently inflate the cuff using the sphygmomanometer. Inflate the cuff an additional 10–20 mmHg beyond the point at which the pulse can no longer be heard.

6 Slowly deflate the cuff and listen carefully for a return of the pulse signal. The systolic blood pressure reading is the pressure at which the pulse can first be clearly heard.

7 Continue deflating the cuff and listen for the point (diastolic pressure) at which the audio signal of the pulse returns to pre-inflation quality. Thereafter completely deflate the cuff.

8 In a conscious animal, 6–8 blood pressure measurements should be taken to ensure reliability. Discard the first measurement if it is very different from the others. Variability in systolic readings should be <20%. Record the mean systolic and diastolic pressures.

Oscillometric technique

This uses a cuff to occlude the artery, and detects oscillations of the underlying artery when it is partly occluded. **This system determines systolic, diastolic and mean arterial pressures.** This method is less accurate in very small patients, patients with low blood pressure and patients with dysrhythmias. Muscle contractions also create oscillations and are a source of potential error.

1 Place the cuff snugly (see Step 4 above) over one of the following:
   - The radial artery proximal to the carpus
   - The saphenous artery proximal to the tarsus
   - The brachial artery proximal to the elbow
   - The median caudal artery at the base of the tail.

2 Attach the cuff to a control unit that continually senses arterial pressure and inflates to a pressure greater than the systolic, and then automatically deflates the cuff.

3 The heart rate is displayed. Verify that this matches the patient's heart rate by manually counting the rate using direct heart auscultation or palpation of an artery.

4 Record the values for 3–5 cycles and report the averages for systolic, diastolic and mean pressures.

Potential false readings

Incorrect blood pressure readings may be obtained due to:

- Inappropriate cuff size
- Inappropriate placement of the cuff
- Excessive motion of the limb or tail
- Low blood pressure
- Dysrhythmias
- Obesity
- Peripheral oedema
- Limb conformation that does not permit snug placement of the cuff
- Stress

Blood sampling – (a) arterial

Indications/Use

- To obtain a sample of arterial blood for assessment of:
    - Respiratory function
    - Arterial oxygen concentration
    - Acid–base status

Contraindications

- Severe coagulopathy
- Sampling should not be performed at sites where the risk of bacterial contamination and infection is high, e.g. due to local tissue damage, local skin infection, diarrhoea, urinary incontinence

Equipment

- A pre-heparinized arterial blood gas syringe with a 23–25 G, $^5/_8$ inch needle attached

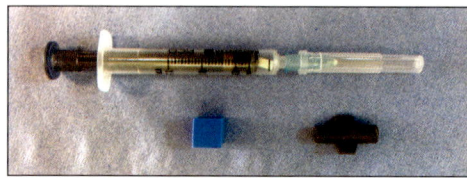

- 70% surgical spirit
- Cotton wool or gauze swabs
- 25 mm wide cohesive bandage (e.g. Vetrap)

Patient preparation and positioning

- Arterial blood sampling is performed in the conscious animal.
- Sedation should be avoided if possible as it will affect test results
- Animals should be positioned appropriately for the blood collection site (see below).

Sites

Most commonly the dorsal pedal artery is used, but in cats and small dogs it is sometimes easier to use the femoral artery.

Dorsal pedal artery

- The animal is placed in lateral recumbency, either on a table (cats and small dogs) or on the floor (large dogs), with the leg to be sampled placed closest to the table or floor.
- An assistant restrains the patient's head with one hand and the uppermost hindlimb with the other.
- The artery is palpated just distal to the tarsus (hock), between the second and third metatarsal bones, on the dorsal aspect.

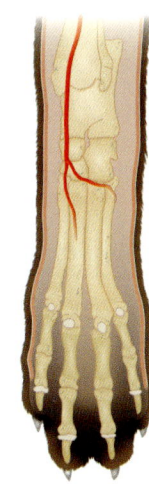

Femoral artery

- The animal is placed in lateral recumbency, either on a table (cats and small dogs) or on the floor (large dogs), with the leg to be sampled placed closest to the table or floor.
- The animal is restrained manually, and the upper limb abducted so that the femoral artery can be palpated.
- The femoral artery pulse is palpable on the medial thigh, ventral to the inguinal region and proximal to the stifle.

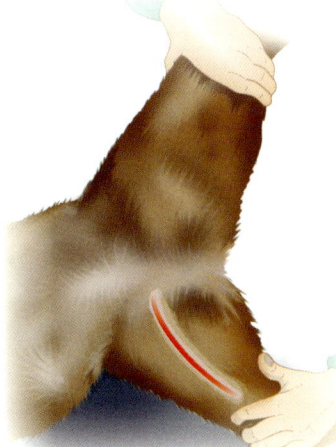

Technique

1. Stretch the skin over the artery.
2. Palpate the artery.
3. The skin overlying the artery is gently clipped, then sprayed or lightly wiped with surgical spirit. Excessive scrubbing/wiping of the skin should be avoided, as this may result in spasm of the artery.
4. Gently rest two fingertips of one hand against the artery, so that the arterial pulse can be felt.

5   With the other hand, direct the needle, with the syringe attached, towards the artery, at an angle of about 30 degrees. The needle bevel is pointed upwards.
6   Penetrate the artery in one quick firm purposeful movement.
7   When the artery has been penetrated, a flash of blood will be seen in the hub of the needle.
8   Collect approximately 1 ml of blood.
9   Remove the syringe and needle from the artery.
10 On removal of the needle, apply direct pressure to the artery for 5 minutes, then cover with cotton wool or a gauze swab and cohesive bandage.
11 Hold the syringe upright and tap it to cause air bubbles to rise. Eject any air from the syringe.
12 Cap the sample with an airtight seal to prevent exposure to room air. Rubber bungs or plastic caps are available with pre-heparinized blood-gas syringes.
13 The blood sample must be analysed as soon as possible, ideally **within 5 minutes**.

APPROXIMATE NORMAL ARTERIAL BLOOD GAS VALUES FOR DOGS AND CATS BREATHING ROOM AIR		
Parameter	Dogs	Cats
pH	7.35–7.46	7.31–7.46
PCO_2	30.8–42.8 mmHg (4.10–5.69 kPa)	25.2–36.8 mmHg (3.35–4.89 kPa)
PO_2	80.9–103.3 mmHg (10.76–13.74 kPa)	95.4–118.2 mmHg (12.69–15.72 kPa)
$[HCO_3^-]$	18.8–25.6 mmol/l	14.4–21.6 mmol/l
Base excess	0 ± 4	0 ± 4

Potential complications

- Significant haemorrhage is very uncommon, provided direct pressure is applied to the artery (see above)
- Bruising and the formation of a small haematoma will occur in some patients, but can be minimized by good technique and by the application of direct pressure to the artery
- Arterial thrombosis and thrombophlebitis are uncommon, but are more likely if repeated attempts are made to collect blood from an artery.

Blood sampling – (b) venous

Indications/Use

- To obtain a sample of venous blood for clinical pathology tests or for bacterial culture

Contraindications

- Coagulopathy
- Sampling should not be performed at sites where risk of bacterial contamination and infection are high, e.g. due to local tissue damage, local skin infection, diarrhoea, urinary incontinence

Equipment

- Hypodermic needles:
  - Cats: 23–21 G; $5/8$ inch
  - Dogs: 21 G; $5/8$ or 1 inch
- 2–10 ml syringes
- 70% surgical spirit
- 4% chlorhexidine gluconate or 10% povidone–iodine
- Cotton wool or gauze swabs
- 25 mm wide cohesive bandage (e.g. Vetrap)
- Appropriate blood containers (see table below) and/or three blood culture bottles (pre-warmed to 37°C)
- Sterile gloves

Additives	Universal *	Vacutainer *	Sample	Tests	Comments
EDTA (ethylene diamine tetra-acetic acid)	Pink/red	Lavender or pink	Whole blood	Haematology	Fill tube precisely to level indicated. Underfilling may cause artefacts; overfilling may lead to clotting
None	White/clear	Red	Serum	Biochemistry; bile acids; serology	
Serum gel	Brown	Gold	Serum	Biochemistry; bile acids; serology	
Lithium heparin	Orange or green	Green or green/ orange	Plasma	Biochemistry; electrolytes	Do not use blood that has been mixed with EDTA
Sodium fluoride and potassium oxalate	Yellow	Grey	Whole blood	Blood glucose	Fluoride/oxalate inhibits red blood cells oxidizing glucose
Sodium citrate	Lilac	Light blue	Whole blood	Coagulation tests; platelet counts	

*Always check cap colour codes, as they may vary with manufacturer

Patient preparation and positioning

- Venous blood sampling is performed in the conscious animal, although in fractious animals light sedation may be required.
- Cats can be wrapped in a large towel to control their limbs when sampling from the jugular vein; for sampling a peripheral vein the target limb can be excluded from the towel.
- The animal should be positioned appropriately for the blood collection site (see below).
- A generous area over the target vein should be clipped, sufficient to allow identification of the vein, and of the direction in which it runs.

REDUCING STRESS

- Many cats and some dogs are frightened by the noise of clippers:
  - Battery-operated models often make less noise and some are specifically designed to be quiet
  - Switch the clippers on at a distance from the animal while talking to it, to mask the initial noise
  - If the animal is fear-aggressive or particularly nervous, consider using a peripheral vein which can be clipped with curved scissors.
- Applying a local anaesthetic cream (e.g. EMLA) or spray (e.g. Intubeaze) to the skin may help to reduce resistance from the animal.

- Using cotton wool or gauze swabs, clean the skin over the vein with 4% chlorhexidine or 10% povidone–iodine, followed by spraying or wiping with surgical spirit.
- When taking samples for bacterial culture, take care not to touch the site of needle insertion. If necessary, gloves should be worn.

Sites

The jugular vein is usually preferred, as it is large enough to allow a sample to be withdrawn rapidly without requiring excessive negative pressure. This minimizes haemolysis and blood clot formation within the sample. The cephalic vein and the lateral saphenous vein may be used: if the jugular vein is not accessible; if the animal resents being restrained for jugular sampling; or if there is a planned procedure that may be compromised by jugular vein haematoma or haemorrhage (e.g. jugular catheter placement or thyroid surgery).

Jugular vein

- The animal is placed in a sitting position, either on a table (cats and small dogs) or on the floor (large dogs).
- An assistant stands on the left of the patient.
- The assistant places their right arm over the patient's back and round the front of the patient, to encircle and control the forelimbs.
- The assistant's left arm is used to extend the animal's neck by grasping its muzzle and directing the nostrils towards the ceiling.

- Fear-aggressive cats, or those that are especially wriggly, can be restrained for jugular sampling by placing them on their side or on their back, controlling the limbs with the hands and body, or wrapping the cat in a towel.
- Raise the vein with one hand by applying gently pressure to the jugular groove at around the level of the jugular inlet.

Cephalic vein

- The animal is placed in a sitting position or in sternal recumbency, either on a table (cats and small dogs) or on the floor (large dogs).
- An assistant stands on the left of the patient.
- The assistant passes their left hand under the patient's neck and holds the head turned away from the sampler.
- The assistant's right arm is used to extend the patient's right forelimb.
- The assistant holding the animal raises the vein by wrapping a thumb around the forelimb just distal to the elbow, and then gently rotating their wrist to encourage the vein onto the cranial aspect of the forelimb.

Lateral saphenous vein

- The animal is placed in lateral recumbency, either on a table (cats and small dogs) or on the floor (large dogs).
- An assistant restrains the animal's head with one hand.
- With the other hand, the assistant extends the uppermost hindlimb, at the same time stretching out the body.
- The assistant holding the animal raises the vein by encircling the caudal aspect of the upper hindlimb, applying pressure at the level of the stifle.

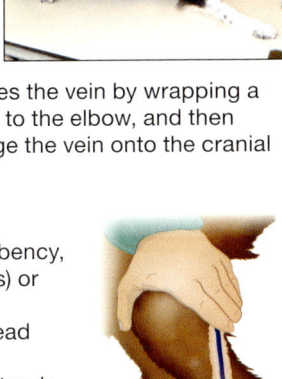

Technique

For biochemical tests or haematology

1 Insert the needle into the vein, with syringe attached and the bevel upwards, at an angle of approximately 30 degrees.
2 Follow the line of the vein with the needle tip.
3 Aspirate blood by applying gentle negative pressure to the syringe plunger. Avoid excessive suction on the syringe, as this may collapse the vein. If no blood is present in the hub, try gently redirecting the needle to enter the vein, but avoid large sweeping movements. If necessary, withdraw the needle and

B

start again with a fresh one.

4   Release the pressure on the vein.

5   Remove the needle. If sampling was from the jugular vein, apply gentle pressure to the venepuncture site for 30–60 seconds. If the cephalic or saphenous vein was used, apply a light bandage of gauze swab or cotton wool held by cohesive bandage for 30–60 minutes.

6   Place the blood sample into the appropriate tube(s).

> ### EDTA TUBES
>
> Blood should be placed in the tube containing EDTA anticoagulant last, as inadvertent contamination of other sample collection tubes with EDTA can adversely affect the results of several biochemical parameters including potassium, calcium and alkaline phosphatase.

7   Gently invert the sample tube several times to ensure adequate distribution of any additive. Do NOT shake the tube, as this may cause haemolysis.

For bacterial culture

1-5 Follow steps 1 to 5 above to take a 5–10 ml blood sample (see culture bottle for required volume). As a relatively large volume of blood is required, the jugular vein should be used.

6   Place a new needle on the syringe.

7   Swab the rubber stopper of the culture bottle with surgical spirit and allow to dry.

8   Add the required volume of blood to the pre-warmed culture bottle.

9   Collect three blood samples with a minimum of 1 hour between samples OR, in acutely septic patients, all three samples can be taken over 30 minutes.

10 The culture bottles should be transported to the laboratory as quickly as possible. Although not ideal, overnight postage may still give meaningful results.

Potential complications

These are very uncommon but may include:

- Minor haemorrhage
- Subcutaneous haematoma formation
- Thrombophlebitis

> ### FURTHER INFORMATION
>
> For information on the interpretation of blood samples see the *BSAVA Manual of Canine and Feline Clinical Pathology*.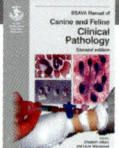

Blood smear preparation

Indications/Use

- Assessment of:
  - White blood cell differential count
  - Leucocyte abnormalities, e.g. toxic neutrophils, left shift, blast cells
  - Red blood cell morphology, e.g. polychromasia, anisocytosis, fragmented cells, spherocytes, Heinz bodies, parasites
  - Platelet count
  - Platelet abnormalities, e.g. macroplatelets, platelet clumps

Equipment

- Fresh blood collected in an EDTA anticoagulant tube (see **Blood sampling – (b) venous**)
- Microhaematocrit tube
- Microscope slides
- A 'spreader' slide: this is narrower than the smear slide to avoid spreading the cells over the edge of the slide. 'Spreaders' can be made by breaking the corner off a normal slide, having first scored it with a blade or diamond writer
- Hairdryer
- Suitable stain (e.g. Diff-Quik)
- Microscope

Technique

Photos from *BSAVA Manual of Feline Practice* and courtesy of Séverine Tasker

1   Invert the EDTA tube several times to make sure the blood is well mixed. Remove a small amount of blood using a microhaemocrit tube held at a near horizontal angle.

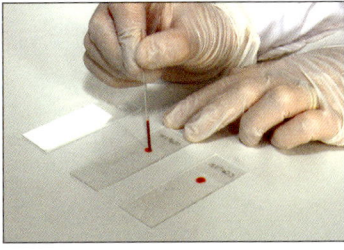

2   Place a small drop of blood on the midline of a microscope slide, towards one end.

3   Hold the 'spreader' between the thumb and middle finger, placing the index finger on top of the 'spreader'.

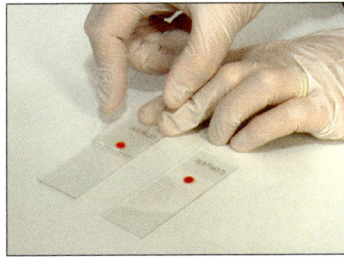

4 Place the 'spreader' in front of the blood spot, at an angle of about 30 degrees, and draw it backwards until it comes into contact with the blood, allowing the blood to spread out rapidly along the edge of the 'spreader'.

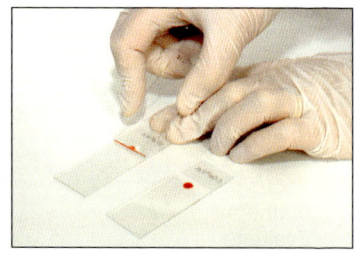

5 The moment this occurs, while keeping the 'spreader' slide at the same angle, move it rapidly yet smoothly away from you to create a blood smear.

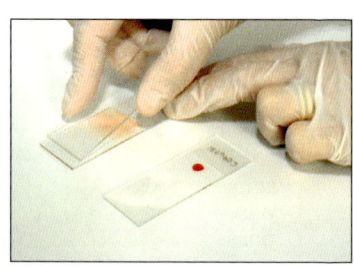

6 As the smear is made, a 'feathered edge' forms. Do not lift the 'spreader' slide until the feathered edge is complete.

7 Ideally, the smear should extend approximately two-thirds of the length of the slide.

8 Rapidly air-dry the blood smear by waving it in the air or using a hairdryer.

9 The smear can be sent to an external laboratory or stained in house with Romanowsky-type stains (e.g. Diff-Quik) for routine examination.

PRACTICAL TIPS: COMMON FAULTS AND HOW TO AVOID THEM

Fault	How to avoid
Film too thick	Use a smaller drop of blood
Film too thin	Use a larger drop of blood and/or faster spreading motion
Alternating thick and thin bands	Ensure spreading motion is smooth and avoid hesitation
Streaks along length of smear	Ensure edge of spreader is not irregular or coated with dried blood Ensure no dust on slide or in blood
'Holes' in smear	Ensure slide is free of grease
Narrow, thick smear	Allow blood to spread right across spreader slide before making smear

Examination

The stained smear is examined using a microscope:

1 Scan the whole smear at low power (X100 total magnification).
2 Examine areas of interest under higher power (X1000, using oil immersion).
3 Focus on the section of the smear (typically just behind the feathered edge) that is composed of a monolayer of cells.
4 Evaluate, in turn: red blood cells, white blood cells, and platelets.

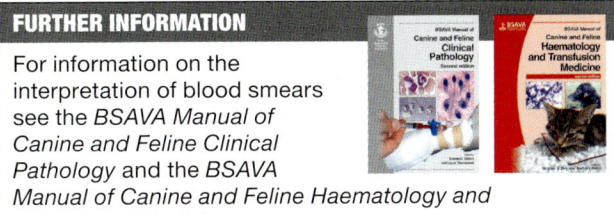

FURTHER INFORMATION

For information on the interpretation of blood smears see the *BSAVA Manual of Canine and Feline Clinical Pathology* and the *BSAVA Manual of Canine and Feline Haematology and Transfusion Medicine*.

Blood transfusion – (a) collection

Donor selection

Changes in guidelines provided by the Royal College of Veterinary Surgeons note that the taking of blood from donors for immediate and anticipated clinical need is a recognized veterinary practice, and the UK Veterinary Medicines Directorate now permits authorization of blood banks for non-food animals following application for a specific licence. These combined changes in legislation and guidance have provided the opportunity for the development of in-house and commercial blood banking in the UK.

Dogs
- Healthy, fully vaccinated, not receiving medication (except routine endo- and ectoparasitic medications)
- Suitable temperament
- >25 kg lean bodyweight
- 1–8 years of age
- Normal PCV, preferably >40%
- Ideally DEA 1.1-negative
- No history of a previous blood transfusion
- Not been vaccinated within the previous 14 days
- No history of travel outside the UK
- Blood can be collected every 8 weeks without the need for iron supplementation

Cats
- Healthy, fully vaccinated, not receiving medication (except routine endo- and ectoparasitic medications)
- Suitable temperament

- >4 kg lean bodyweight
- 1–8 years of age
- PCV >35%
- Blood typed (A, B or AB)
- No history of a previous blood transfusion
- No history of travel outside the UK
- Negative for FeLV and FIV as evaluated by a standard in-house ELISA technique
- Negative for haemotropic *Mycoplasma* spp. evaluated by PCR
- Blood can be collected every 8 weeks without the need for iron supplementation

Equipment

- As required for **Aseptic preparation – (a) non-surgical procedures**
- Blood collection containers:
    - *Dogs:* standard commercial blood collection bag containing an anticoagulant, such as citrate phosphate dextrose (CPD), citrate phosphate dextrose adenine (CPDA) or acid citrate dextrose (ACD), attached to an extension tube and a swaged-on 16 G phlebotomy needle. These closed systems are much preferred to open systems due to the reduced potential for bacterial contamination and thus a prolonged shelf life
    - *Cats:* Three 20 ml syringes prefilled with anticoagulant (1 ml CPD, CPDA or ACD per 7.3 ml blood), a 19 or 21 G butterfly catheter or 19 G needle, 3-way tap, short extension tubing and capped needles or syringe caps
- Topical local anaesthetic cream (e.g. EMLA cream)
- Electronic scales (for weighing blood collection bags)
- Artery forceps
- Gauze swabs
- Clamping device and clamps
- Materials for a light neck bandage

Patient preparation and positioning

- Ensure that the donor meets the criteria listed above.
- Most dogs are able to donate blood without being sedated. Cats typically require sedation.

EXAMPLES OF FELINE DONOR SEDATION PROTOCOLS

- Ketamine 5 mg/kg and midazolam 0.25 mg/kg i.m. given together in the same syringe. Two separate doses of this sedative combination are prepared in advance; the second dose can be given as a 'top-up' intravenously (in 0.05–0.1 ml increments) as required.
- Butorphanol 0.1–0.2 mg/kg ± diazepam 0.5 mg/kg i.v.
- Ketamine 2 mg/kg and midazolam 0.1 mg/kg i.v.; additional boluses of one-quarter to one-half of the original dose as required.
- Mask isoflurane/oxygen anaesthesia.

- If required, apply topical local anaesthetic cream at least 20 minutes prior to the procedure.
- Restrain dogs securely in lateral recumbency or in a sitting position on a table.
- Restrain cats on their back with the neck extended for optimal visualization of the jugular vein; either side of the neck can be used. Alternatively, restrain the cat in lateral recumbency with the neck outstretched.

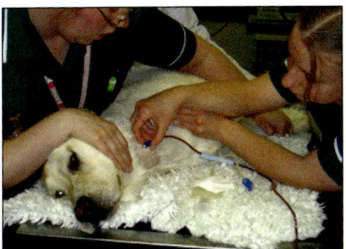
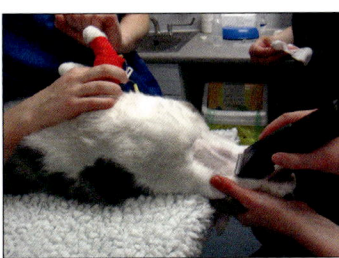

- In cats, it is advisable to preplace an **intravenous catheter** in a cephalic vein for the purpose of administering intravenous fluids following blood donation
- **Aseptic preparation – (a) non-surgical procedures** is carried out on the skin overlying the jugular groove.

Collection procedure

Dogs

1 An assistant applies gentle pressure at the thoracic inlet to raise the jugular vein. Avoid contamination of the venepuncture site.
2 Remove the needle cap and perform venepuncture using the 16 G phlebotomy needle attached to the collection bag. If no flashback of blood is seen in the tubing, check needle placement and tubing for occlusion. The needle may need to be repositioned, but should not be fully withdrawn from the patient.
3 Position the bag lower than the donor to aid in gravitational flow and on a set of electronic scales.
4 Periodically invert the bag to ensure adequate mixing of blood and anticoagulant.
5 The maximum canine donation volume is approximately 16–18 ml/kg. The volume of blood that should be collected into a commercial blood bag is 450 ml, with an allowable 10% variance (405–495 ml). The weight of 1 ml of canine blood is approximately 1.053 g; therefore, the weight of an acceptable unit using one of these bags is approximately 426–521 g.
6 When the bag is full, clamp the tubing with a pair of artery forceps and remove the needle from the jugular vein.
7 Using a gauze swab, apply pressure over the venepuncture site for 5 minutes. A light neck bandage should be applied for several hours.
8 Strip any blood remaining in the tubing into the bag, using the fingers, inverting the bag several times to ensure adequate

mixing. Allow the tubing to refill with anticoagulant blood and clamp the distal (needle) end with a hand sealer clip or heat sealer. If these are not available, a knot can be tied in the line, although this is less desirable.

9 Clamp the entire length of tubing into 10 cm segments to be used for **cross-matching**.

10 Label the bag with the product type, donor identification, date of collection, date of expiration, donor blood type, donor PVC and phlebotomist identification prior to use or storage.

11 Following donation, food and water can be offered. Activity should be restricted to lead walks only for the next 24 hours, and it is advised that a harness or lead passed under the chest is used instead of a neck collar and lead, to avoid pressure on the jugular venepuncture site.

Cats

1 Attach a syringe to one port of the 3-way tap and a butterfly catheter or 21 G needle to another port. A short extension tube can be attached between the 3-way tap and the butterfly catheter if required.

2 Flush the tubing with anticoagulant solution.

3 An assistant applies pressure at the thoracic inlet to raise the jugular vein. Avoid contamination of the venepuncture site.

4 Perform venepuncture using the butterfly catheter or 21 G needle. Without removing the butterfly catheter, perform venepuncture and fill each syringe in turn. The syringes can be rocked gently to ensure adequate mixing of blood and anticoagulant during collection.

5 When each syringe has been filled, close the 3-way tap, remove the syringe and place a capped needle or syringe cap on the end.

6 The maximum feline donation volume is approximately 11–13 ml/kg. When the required amount of blood has been collected, remove the butterfly needle from the vein.

7 Using a gauze swab, apply pressure over the venepuncture site for 5 minutes. A light neck bandage can be applied for several hours.

8 Label each syringe with the donor identification, blood type, time of collection and phlebotomist identification.

9 During or immediately after blood collection, 100 ml of an intravenous crystalloid should be given via the cephalic vein over 1–2 hours. The donor must be closely observed during recovery and may be offered food and water once fully awake. The donor can usually be discharged after 8–12 hours. Remove the neck bandage before sending the cat home and check the venepuncture site for bleeding.

Potential complications

- Haematoma
- Hypovolaemic shock

Storage

- Whole blood collected in a bag should be stored in a refrigerator maintained at 1–6°C with the bag in an upright position. Positioning the bag in this manner maximizes gas exchange with the red cell solution to help preserve the viability of the red blood cells during storage and following transfusion.
- Whole blood collected in a bag should be used within 28 days.
- Blood collected using an open system, e.g. into syringes, should be administered within 4 hours, or refrigerated and used within 24 hours.
- Whole blood can also be separated into packed red blood cells, fresh plasma, stored plasma and platelet-rich plasma concentrates. This should be done as soon as possible after collection, and plasma should be frozen within 8 hours to preserve coagulation and anticoagulation factors (fresh frozen plasma).

Blood transfusion – (b) cross-matching

Indications/Use

- To determine serological compatibility between a patient and donor blood

Dogs

Cross-matching should be performed whenever:

- The recipient has received a blood transfusion >4 days previously, even if a DEA 1.1-negative donor was used
- There has been a history of transfusion reaction
- The recipient's transfusion history is unknown
- The recipient has had puppies

Cats

Cross-matching should be performed whenever:

- The recipient requires more than one transfusion, as previously transfused blood (even though it was the same AB type) may induce antibody production against red blood cell antigens separate from the AB blood group
- The donor or recipient blood type is unknown.

Equipment

- Approximately 5 ml of blood collected in an EDTA anticoagulant tube from both the donor and recipient
- Centrifuge
- 5 ml plain plastic tubes
- 0.9% saline
- Pipette
- Microscope slides
- Microscope

Patient preparation and positioning

See **Blood sampling – (b) venous**

Technique

1   Collect blood from the jugular veins of the donor *and* recipient. Approximately 5 ml of blood from each should be placed into separate EDTA tubes (see **Blood sampling – (b) venous**). Alternatively, a sample of anticoagulated blood from the clamped sections of tubing of the blood collection bag (dogs) or collection syringes (cats) can be used.

2   Centrifuge the tubes (usually at 1000 RPM for 5–10 minutes), remove the supernatants (plasma) and transfer them to clean labelled 5 ml plain tubes (donor and recipient) for later use.

3   If a centrifuge is not available, allow the EDTA tubes to stand for ≥1 hour until the red blood cells have settled before using the supernatant.

Standard cross-match procedure

1   Wash the red blood cells three times with 0.9% saline and discard the supernatant after each wash.

2   Resuspend the washed red blood cells to create a 3–5% solution by adding 0.2 ml of red blood cells to 4.8 ml of saline (1 drop of red blood cells to 20 drops of saline).

3   For each donor prepare three tubes labelled as major, minor and recipient control.

4   To each tube add 1 drop of the appropriate 3–5% red blood cells and 2 drops of plasma according to the following:

   i   Major cross-match = donor red blood cells and recipient plasma

   ii   Minor cross-match = recipient red blood cells and donor plasma

   iii Recipient control = recipient red blood cells and recipient plasma.

5   Incubate the tubes for 15 minutes at room temperature.

6   Centrifuge the tubes at 1000 RPM for approximately 15 seconds to allow the cells to settle. Examine the samples for haemolysis (reddening of the supernatant).

7   Gently tap the tubes to resuspend the cells. Examine and score the tubes for agglutination.

8   If macroscopic agglutination is not observed, transfer a small amount of the tube contents to a labelled glass slide and examine for microscopic agglutination. This should not be confused with rouleaux formation (see **Haemagglutination**).

9   For the recipient control:

   i   If there is no haemolysis or agglutination in the recipient control tube, the results are valid and incompatibilities can be interpreted

   ii   If there is haemolysis or agglutination present in the recipient control tube, then the compatibility and suitability of the donor cannot be accurately assessed.

Rapid slide cross-match procedure

An alternative and more rapid, but potentially less accurate, procedure for cross-match analysis involves visualizing the presence of agglutination on a slide rather than in a tube.

1 For each donor prepare three slides labelled as major, minor and recipient control.

2 Place 1 drop of red blood cells and 2 drops of plasma on to each slide according to the following:
- **i** Major cross-match = donor red blood cells and recipient plasma
- **ii** Minor cross-match = recipient red blood cells and donor plasma
- **iii** Recipient control = recipient red blood cells and recipient plasma.

3 Gently rock the slides to mix the plasma and red blood cells. Examine for agglutination after 1–5 minutes.

4 For the recipient control: agglutination will invalidate results.

Results of cross-matching

- Any agglutination and/or haemolysis is a 'positive' result.
- A positive **recipient control** indicates that the patient is autoagglutinating. This makes interpretation of the test difficult, although it can be repeated with additional washing of the recipient's red blood cells.
- A positive **major cross-match** indicates a significant antibody titre in the recipient against the donor red blood cells and **precludes the use of that donor for transfusions**.
- A positive **minor cross-match** indicates the presence of antibodies in the donor against the recipient red blood cells. If this reaction is strong, even small volumes of donor plasma may cause a significant transfusion reaction and precludes the use of the donor (unless red blood cells can be washed). With a weaker reaction, packed red blood cells from the donor may be transfused.

> **WARNING**
>
> - **Despite using blood products from a cross-match-compatible donor, it is still possible for a patient to experience a haemolytic or non-haemolytic transfusion reaction. Recipient monitoring during and following administration of blood products is essential.**

Blood transfusion – (c) typing

Indications/Use

- **Dogs:** As DEA 1.1 is the most antigenic blood type, it is strongly advised that the DEA 1.1 status of both the donor and recipient is

- determined prior to transfusion, or that only DEA 1.1-negative donors are used
- **Cats: All donor and recipient cats must be blood typed** prior to transfusion, even in an emergency situation

Equipment

- Approximately 2 ml of blood collected into an EDTA tube (see **Blood sampling – (b) venous**)
- Blood can be submitted to a commercial laboratory for typing
- *Alternatively*, two different commercial kits are available for in-house typing

Dogs

- Rapid Vet-H test: This is a test card with three test 'wells' used for determining whether a dog is DEA 1.1 +ve or –ve. Two wells contain anti-DEA 1.1 antibodies, and there is also a 'control' well containing no anti-DEA 1.1 reagent. Interpretation is based on looking for the presence or absence of agglutination in the patient test well.
- Quick Test DEA1.1: This migration paper strip cartridge uses monoclonal antibodies to determine whether a dog is DEA 1.1 +ve or –ve. A line adjacent to the DEA 1.1 line and the control line indicates that the dog is positive for this blood group.

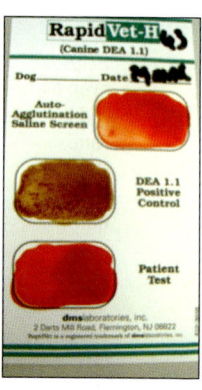

Cats

- Rapid Vet-H test: This is a test card with three test 'wells': the type A well contains anti-type A reagent; the type B well contains anti-type B reagent; there is also a 'control' well containing no anti-A or anti-B reagents. Interpretation is based on looking for an agglutination reaction in either or both test wells.

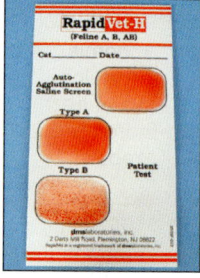

- Quick Test A+B: This migration paper strip cartridge uses monoclonal antibodies to differentiate blood types. A line adjacent to the relevant blood group (A or B) and the control line (C) indicates the cat's blood group.

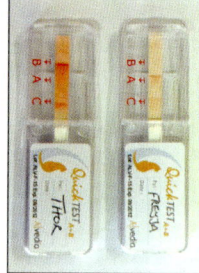

Patient preparation and positioning

See **Blood sampling – (b) venous**

Technique

Use a commercial blood typing test kit and follow manufacturer's instructions.

Blood transfusion – (d) giving

Indications/Use

- Anaemia
- Coagulopathies, although consideration should be given to the use of fresh frozen plasma or cryoprecipitate. Note, however, that stored blood will be severely depleted in several clotting factors
- Preparation for anticipated blood loss during surgery

Contraindications

- Administration of non-typed or non-cross-matched blood to a dog that has previously received a blood transfusion
- Administration of non-typed blood to a cat

Equipment

- As required for **Intravenous catheter placement**

- Whole blood:
  - **Dogs:** As a general rule:
    - DEA 1.1-negative dogs should *only* receive DEA 1.1-negative blood
    - DEA 1.1-positive dogs may receive *either* DEA 1.1-negative or -positive blood

- **Cats:**
  - Type A cats must *only* receive type A blood
  - Type B cats must *only* receive type B blood
  - The rarer type AB cats do not possess either alloantibody; they should ideally receive type AB blood, but when this is not available type A blood is the next best choice, followed by type B blood

---

INSPECTION OF BLOOD

Visual inspection of the blood is necessary prior to administration. Discoloration (brown, purple), the presence of clots or haemolysis may indicate bacterial contamination and the blood should not be used.

- **Dogs:** Blood infusion set incorporating an in-line filter (170–260 μm) and suitable for connecting to a canine blood collection bag
- **Cats:** A plain 150 ml blood collection bag and blood giving set with in-line filter (170–260 μm). All the blood collected into the syringes is injected slowly into the plain blood collection bag through the injection port

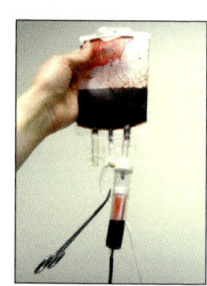

Alternatively, blood collected into syringes can be administered via an extension set using a syringe driver. Again a filter should be used, such as a paediatric filter with reduced dead space or microaggregate filters of 18–40 μm

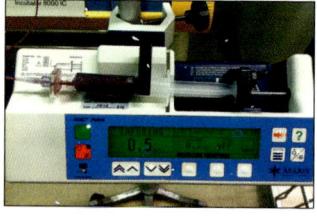

- Intravenous catheter suitable for the size of the patient. A large-diameter catheter should be placed to avoid red cell haemolysis during blood administration
- Adhesive tape

Patient preparation and positioning

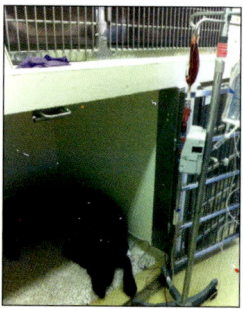

- The patient should ideally be conscious, although sedation can be used if required. It is sometimes necessary to give blood to an anaesthetized patient intraoperatively.
- The patient should be placed on comfortable bedding.

- Patients should not receive food or medication during a transfusion, and the only fluid that may be administered through the same catheter is 0.9% saline.
- An **intravenous catheter** should be placed in a peripheral vein. *Alternatively,* blood can be given via an **intraosseous cannula** if venous access cannot be obtained.

Technique

> **NOTES**
>
> - Blood is usually administered intravenously via an intravenous catheter, but it may also be given via the intraosseous route if venous access cannot be obtained (e.g. kittens, puppies). It should *not* be given intraperitoneally.
> - Blood does not need to be warmed prior to use, unless being given to neonates or other very small animals. Warming may lead to haemolysis of red cells, as well as providing favourable conditions for proliferation of any microbial contaminant.
> - Care should be taken if blood is administered to patients with increased risk of volume overload (e.g. cardiovascular disease, impaired renal function).
> - Blood should not be given through a catheter that contains, or has contained without flushing, calcium-containing fluids (e.g. Hartmann's (lactated Ringer's) solution, Ringer's solution, some colloids).

Volume

The amount of blood to be administered can be calculated as follows:

- As a 'rule of thumb':
    - 2 ml blood/kg bodyweight raises the PCV by 1%
- Suggested formulae for calculating the amount of whole blood required for transfusion are:

DOG:

Volume of donor blood required =

recipient's bodyweight (kg) x 85 x $\dfrac{\text{desired PCV} - \text{recipient's PCV}}{\text{PCV of donated blood}}$

CAT:

Volume of donor blood required =

recipient's bodyweight (kg) x 60 x $\dfrac{\text{desired PCV} - \text{recipient's PCV}}{\text{PCV of donated blood}}$

- **Total volume given should not exceed 22 ml/kg unless there are severe ongoing losses.**

Rate

The rate of whole blood administration depends on the cardiovascular status of the recipient:

- In general, the rate should be only 0.25–1.0 ml/kg/h for the first 20–30 minutes
- If the transfusion is well tolerated, the rate may then be increased to around 5–10 ml/kg/h, aiming to deliver the remaining product within 4 hours. *Blood should not be administered over a period longer than 4 hours owing to the increased risk of bacterial proliferation within the product*
- In an animal with an increased risk of volume overload (cardiovascular disease, impaired renal function), the rate of administration should not exceed 3–4 ml/kg/h.

WARNING

- Fluid pumps should NOT be used for RBC transfusions unless they have been validated appropriately for such use by the manufacturer, because they could induce red cell haemolysis.

Monitoring

Continuous monitoring during the transfusion is required for signs of a reaction.

- The following parameters should be recorded prior to the transfusion ('baseline'), every 5 minutes during the first 30 minutes of the transfusion, and then every 15 minutes for the remainder of the transfusion:
  - Demeanour
  - Rectal temperature
  - Pulse rate and quality
  - Respiratory rate and character (see **Cardiorespiratory examination**)
  - Mucous membrane colour and capillary refill time
  - Plasma and urine colour.
- PCV and TP should also be monitored prior to, upon completion of, and at 12 and 24 hours after transfusion.

Adverse reactions and action required

Acute haemolytic reaction with intravascular haemolysis

- Seen in type B cats receiving type A blood, as well as in DEA 1.1-negative dogs sensitized to DEA 1.1 upon repeated exposure.
- Clinical signs may include fever, tachycardia, dyspnoea, muscle tremors, vomiting, weakness, collapse, haemoglobinaemia and haemoglobinuria.
- May lead to shock, disseminated intravascular coagulation, renal damage and, potentially, death.

- **Treatment involves immediate discontinuation of the transfusion** and treatment of the clinical signs of shock.

Non-haemolytic immunological reactions

- Acute type I hypersensitivity reactions (allergic or anaphylactic), most often mediated by IgE and mast cells.
- Clinical signs including urticaria, pruritus, erythema, oedema, vomiting and dyspnoea secondary to pulmonary oedema.
- **Treatment involves immediate discontinuation of the transfusion** and evaluation of the patient for evidence of haemolysis and shock. Steroids (dexamethasone 0.5–1.0 mg/kg i.v.) and antihistamines (chlorphenamine 4–8 mg q8h for dogs; 2–4 mg q8–12h for cats) may be required.

Bone biopsy – needle core

Indications/Use

- To obtain a sample of bone in suspected cases of:
  - Primary bone tumours
  - Metastatic bone tumour
  - Bacterial osteomyelitis
  - Mycosis
- To obtain a bone marrow core biopsy sample

Contraindications

- Coagulopathy
- Fracture in the region to be sampled

Equipment

- Jamshidi bone biopsy needle:
  - 12 G for dogs >5 kg
  - 14 G for dogs <5 kg and cats
- As required for **Aseptic preparation – (a) non-surgical procedures**
- Scalpel
- Tissue glue or suture materials for skin closure
- Container of 10% neutral buffered formalin
- Plain sterile tube for culture (if required)

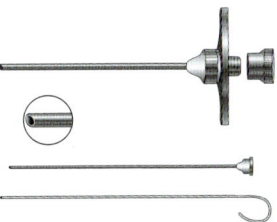

Jamshidi needle

Patient preparation and positioning

- General anaesthesia is essential for both dogs and cats.
- Position the animal with the area to be sampled uppermost:
  - In cases of suspected tumour, bacterial osteomyelitis or mycosis, the centre of the lesion should be sampled, as sampling the periphery will often yield only samples of the reactive bone surrounding the primary lesion. The centre of the lesion is identified by radiography or another diagnostic imaging modality

- When collecting a bone marrow core biopsy sample, the anatomical site for needle insertion is the same as for **bone marrow aspiration**. However, if following bone marrow aspiration, insertion at a slightly different point (on the same limb) or on the contralateral limb is preferable.
- **Aseptic preparation – (a) non-surgical procedures** is performed at the site on an area approximately 10 cm x 10 cm centred on the point of needle insertion.

Technique

1 Make a small skin incision with a scalpel blade over the site of needle insertion.

2 With the stylet of the Jamshidi needle in place, advance the cannula through the soft tissues until the bone is reached.

3 Remove the stylet and penetrate the bone cortex with the cannula, using steady and very firm pressure with clockwise and anticlockwise drilling movements in one plane, with the needle remaining perpendicular.

4 Advance the cannula a sufficient distance into the bone (1–3 cm) such that the lumen of the needle is filled with a core of bone.

5 Section the core of bone from its source at the distal tip of the needle by rotating and moving the handle of the bone marrow needle vigorously in different directions (circular motion and side to side), and then twisting the needle within the bone clockwise a few times and then anticlockwise. These movements should be performed with reasonable force to ensure the core will not be left behind when the needle is withdrawn.

6 Remove the cannula.

7 Insert the blunt probe retrograde into the tip of the cannula to expel the specimen through the handle end. This is important as the cannula tapers towards the free end.

8 Place the specimen into an appropriate collection pot.

9 **If obtaining a sample in cases of suspected tumour, bacterial osteomyelitis or mycosis, it is very important to repeat the procedure with redirection of the needle to obtain multiple core samples.**

10 The skin incision should be sutured or closed with tissue adhesive.

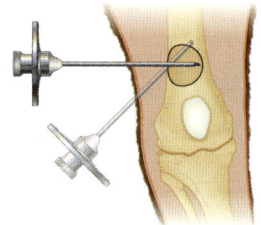

Sample handling

- The sample should be fixed in 10% neutral buffered formalin.
- The sample should be sent to a histopathology laboratory. **NB** The sample will have to be decalcified at the laboratory, a process that may take several days.
- In cases of suspected bacterial osteomyelitis or mycosis, an additional sample should be placed in a sterile plain tube and submitted to the laboratory.

Potential complications

- It is possible that bacterial or fungal infections may spread into the surrounding soft tissue during bone biopsy
- Rarely, bone can be weakened enough for a fracture to occur. This is more likely to happen if multiple samples are taken

Bone marrow aspiration

Indications/Use

To obtain a sample of bone marrow for cytology to aid diagnosis/ staging in:

- Non-regenerative anaemia
- Neutropenia or thrombocytopenia
- Unexplained leucocytosis, polycythaemia or thrombocytosis
- Excessive numbers of cells with abnormal morphology in the peripheral blood
- Pyrexia of unknown origin
- Hyperproteinaemia associated with a monoclonal or polyclonal gammopathy
- Unexplained hypercalcaemia
- Multicentric lymphoma

SAMPLING OPTIONS

- Two types of bone marrow sample are collected for diagnostic purposes:
  - A bone marrow aspirate provides cytological (morphological) information on individual cells;
  - A bone marrow core biopsy (see **Bone biopsy – needle core**) allows evaluation of the degree of cellularity and presence or absence of infiltration with fat or fibrous tissue.
- Ideally, both should be collected, but sometimes presence of bone marrow disease makes sample collection difficult and only one type of sample can be obtained.

Contraindications

- Coagulopathy
- Fracture in the region to be sampled

Equipment

- As required for **Aseptic preparation – (a) non-surgical procedures**
- Klima or Rosenthal needle with interlocking stylet are the author's [NB] preferred needles for collection of a bone marrow aspirate:
    - 14 G for most dogs
    - 16 G for dogs <5 kg and cats

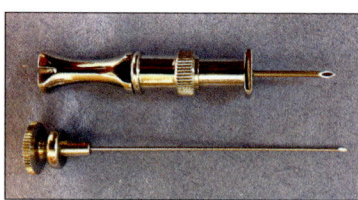
Klima needle

- *Alternatively,* a Jamshidi bone biopsy needle can be used:
    - 12 G for dogs >5 kg
    - 14 G for dogs <5 kg and cats
- 20 ml syringe
- Approximately 1 ml of ACD (acid citrate dextrose) removed from a blood transfusion collection bag

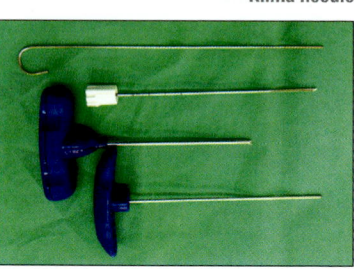
Jamshidi needle

- Local anaesthetic
- Scalpel
- 10–12 clean microscope slides laid out
- Hairdryer
- EDTA collection tube
- Container of 10% neutral buffered formalin (for submission of a small core biopsy sample, if obtained)
- Tissue glue or suture materials for skin closure

PRACTICAL TIP

To prevent the bone marrow clotting, anticoagulant can be drawn up into the 20 ml syringe to coat the entire barrel, and then removed from the syringe while flushing the bone marrow needle with the stylet removed. The stylet should then be replaced in the bone marrow needle.

Patient preparation and positioning

- In dogs, sedation and local anaesthesia are usually sufficient, although the more inexperienced clinician may prefer general anaesthesia.
- In cats, general anaesthesia should be used.
- At least one assistant is necessary, to aid with positioning the animal for correct needle insertion and also to help with making smears of the bone marrow.

- **Aseptic preparation – (a) non-surgical procedures** is performed on an area approximately 10 cm x 10 cm centred on the point of needle insertion.
- Infiltrate 1–2 ml of local anaesthetic into the skin, subcutis and periosteum. Consider the use of a long-acting local anaesthetic to provide analgesia following the procedure.

Technique

1   Make a small stab incision in the skin over the required site:
  - **Dogs:** Iliac crest; greater tubercle of humerus; or trochanteric fossa of the femur
  - **Cats:** Greater tubercle of humerus; or trochanteric fossa of the femur.
2   Introduce a Klima, Rosenthal or Jamshidi bone biopsy needle with the stylet in place, through the skin and subcutis and on to the bone.

Iliac crest (wings of the ilium): Place the animal in sternal recumbency with both hindlimbs pushed tightly under the body.

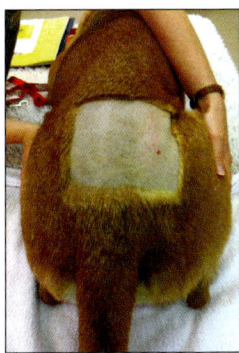

Insert the needle into the widest and most dorsal aspect of the iliac crest. The needle should be aimed down the centre of the iliac crest, which can be found by placing a finger on either side of the bone or by gently redirecting the needle off either side of the bone. The needle should be directed slightly caudally, and remain approximately perpendicular to the skin during insertion.

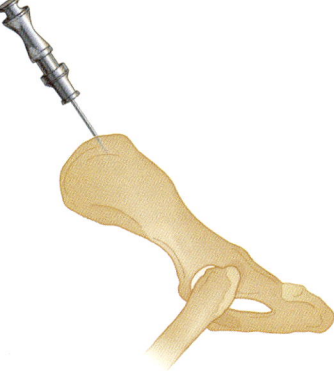

B

Humerus: With the patient in lateral recumbency, insert the needle into the greater tubercle of the proximal humerus and align it with the long axis (shaft) of the humerus.

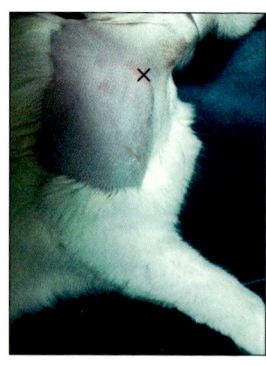

Alternatively, in medium to large dogs, the needle can be inserted on the craniolateral flattened aspect of the proximal humerus, perpendicular to the long axis of the bone. The needle insertion point is made more accessible if an assistant rotates the elbow medially; this limb position should be maintained at all times.

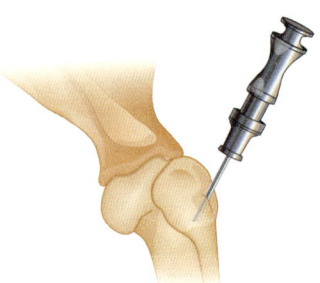

Femur: With the patient in lateral recumbency, palpate the greater trochanter and insert the needle medial to this and into the trochanteric fossa. Once the needle is in the trochanteric fossa, advance it parallel to the long axis (shaft) of the femur. The needle insertion point is made more accessible if an assistant stabilizes the femur by grasping the stifle and applies slight internal (medial) rotation.

> **WARNING**
>
> - It is important to remember that the sciatic nerve is located caudal to the femur and can be damaged if the needle slips caudal to the femur. Sciatic nerve damage can be avoided by walking the needle off the medial edge of the greater trochanter.

3 Gradually advance the needle using steady and very firm pressure with a drilling action (clockwise and anticlockwise movements in one plane, with the needle perpendicular) until the needle enters the medullary cavity. Entry into the

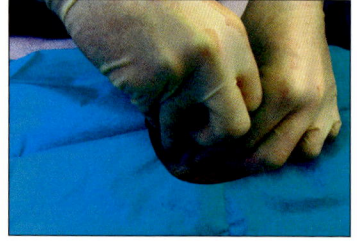

medullary cavity is detected as a decrease in resistance to cannula insertion into the bone, or increased stability of the cannula within the bone. When the cannula is properly seated within the medullary cavity, movement of the cannula will result in the same movement of the bone.

4   Remove the stylet and attach a 20 ml syringe to the needle.

5   Aspirate with several quite forceful withdrawals of the plunger (to around the 10 ml mark on the syringe).

6   Release the plunger as soon as any blood-coloured material appears in the hub of the syringe. Bone marrow aspirate samples usually comprise <0.5 ml.

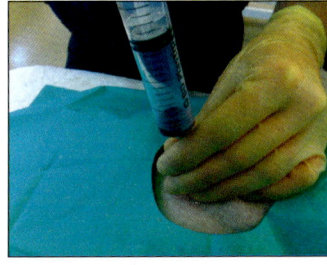

7   Remove the syringe, leaving the needle in place.

8   Immediately process the bone marrow sample, as detailed below.

9   If no bone marrow is obtained this may be due to poor needle placement or to marrow fibrosis. Replace the stylet and advance the needle a further 0.5 cm; then remove the stylet and reapply suction. If this is still not successful, withdraw the needle, replace the stylet and redirect the needle. When two or three attempts have been unsuccessful, an alternative site should be found.

10   *Optional:* After obtaining marrow, the needle may be left in place without the syringe. It can then sometimes be used to obtain a small core biopsy sample, by advancing it a further 10–20 mm into the marrow cavity, without the stylet in place. Rotate the needle vigorously in one direction and then remove it. The core sample is removed from the needle using a blunt probe or, if not available, the stylet. However, **bone biopsy – needle core** is the preferred method for obtaining a core sample.

11   Close the skin deficit with tissue glue or a single suture.

Sample handling

■   Prior to aspiration, place 10–20 clean microscope slides at a near-vertical angle.

■   Place a drop of marrow at the top end of each slide. Excessive blood present in the marrow sample runs down to the bottom of the slide, whilst the marrow spicules should remain at the top of the slide.

■   Smears of the marrow spicules should be made using the squash preparation technique (see **Fine needle aspiration**). Smears should be made quickly, as the marrow clots rapidly (usually within 10–20 seconds). Dry the smears by waving them in the air or by using a hairdryer.

- Unstained smears should be submitted to a laboratory for analysis.
- Excess marrow can be placed in an EDTA tube for cytological evaluation, although morphology will be adversely affected over time.
- If a core biopsy sample is obtained, place this in 10% neutral buffered formalin.

Potential complications

- Significant haemorrhage is unlikely. However, in a severely thrombocytopenic patient, prolonged digital pressure should be applied to the biopsy site
- Puncture or laceration of muscles and nerves

FURTHER INFORMATION

Details of the cytological evaluation of bone marrow are given in the *BSAVA Manual of Canine and Feline Haematology and Transfusion Medicine and the BSAVA Manual of Canine and Feline Clinical Pathology.*

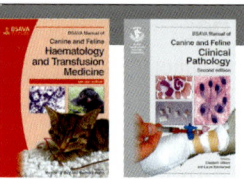

Bronchoalveolar lavage

Indications/Use

- To investigate coughing and suspected bronchial or alveolar disease
- To obtain a sample for cytology and bacteriology from the lower airways of dogs and cats

---

OPTIONS

- Bronchoalveolar lavage (BAL) is used to sample smaller airways (lower bronchioles and alveoli) and can be performed using an endoscope or 'blind'.
- The upper airways of medium and large-sized dogs may also be sampled by **transtracheal wash**.
- The upper airways of dogs and cats may be sampled by **endotracheal wash**.

Contraindications

- Patient not stable enough to undergo anaesthesia (e.g. severe hypoxaemia, cardiac arrhythmia/dysfunction)
- Coagulopathy
- Partial tracheal obstruction
- Unstable asthma
- Pulmonary hypertension

Equipment

- As for **Bronchoscopy** (if performed using a bronchoscope)
- A sterile bronchoalveolar lavage catheter (6 Fr, 124 cm long, with an end rather than a side hole) or a soft urinary catheter (6–8 Fr, 30–60 cm long, with an end hole)
- 500 ml warm 0.9% sterile saline
- 5–20 ml syringes
- Hypodermic needles: 21 G
- Microscope slides
- EDTA and sterile plain collection tubes

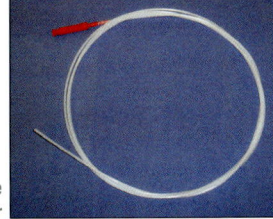

Lavage catheter

Patient preparation and positioning

- Inhalation anaesthesia is generally recommended, although intravenous anaesthesia may be used. An elbow port connector can be used to provide constant gas anaesthesia when performing BAL.
- Pre-oxygenation is very helpful, especially when there is compromised oxygenation. This can be provided through **nasal oxygen delivery** or a face mask. Supplementary oxygen can also be delivered through the channel of the endoscope or via a catheter placed alongside the endoscope. Flow volumes of 1–3 litres per minute can be safely used.
- Position the patient in sternal recumbency with the head elevated and neck extended.
- A mouth gag is essential to keep the mouth open.

> **WARNING**
>
> - **When performing BAL with the aid of a bronchoscope, or performing BAL in a cat, please note the WARNINGS and SPECIAL CONSIDERATIONS detailed in Bronchoscopy.**

Technique

1. If using a bronchoscope, perform **Bronchoscopy**.
2. Once the lung lobes to be sampled have been selected, pass the bronchoscope into successively smaller airways until it sits snugly.
3. Pre-draw sterile saline into several syringes.
4. Instil sterile saline via the biopsy channel of the endoscope:
   - A bolus of 20 ml is used in dogs >10 kg
   - A bolus of 5 ml is used in dogs <10 kg and in cats.
5. Immediately suck the saline back from the biopsy channel using a syringe.
6. Negative pressure during aspiration indicates the need to decrease suction to avoid airway collapse. If necessary, the bronchoscope can be repositioned slightly, taking care not to dislodge the tip of the bronchoscope from the airway in which it is wedged.

7 If air fills the syringe it should be eliminated and additional suction attempts made.

8 Repeat steps 4 to 6 a maximum of 3 times until an adequate sample has been obtained.

9 Ideally, at least two lung lobes should be sampled.

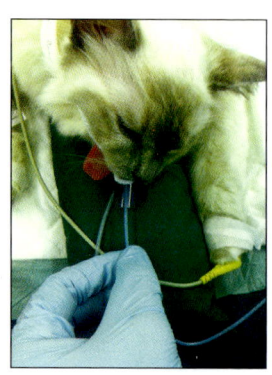

Alternatively, the procedure can be performed using a lavage catheter passed through the biopsy channel of the endoscope.

Alternatively, although this is less preferred, the procedure can be performed 'blind' using a lavage catheter or soft urinary catheter passed without endoscopic assistance. Gently introduce the catheter aseptically into the endotracheal tube (ET) until resistance is felt; at this point the catheter should be lodged within a distal airway. Sterile saline is then instilled and re-aspirated as described above.

NOTES

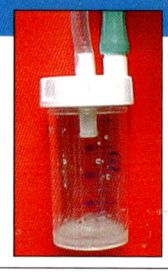

- A total recovery of 40–90% of the instilled volume of saline represents good sample recovery. Recovered fluid is typically slightly turbid, with a foamy layer at the top (representative of surfactant).
- Performing coupage during the procedure may assist sample retrieval.

---

10 Following BAL, continue administration of 100% oxygen and volatile agent for 5 minutes, to allow time to detect any immediate complications, e.g. bronchospasm. Continue oxygen supplementation via the ET tube until extubation. Pulse oximetry should be utilized to measure the patient's oxygenation throughout the recovery from anaesthesia, and during the postoperative period.

Sample handling

- Submit a portion of the sample in a sterile plain tube or culture.
- Place an aliquot in an EDTA tube for cytology.
- The cells collected are fragile, so samples should be processed as soon as possible. If samples are to be sent to an external laboratory, fresh air-dried unstained smears of any flocculent/mucoid material should also be made (see **Fine needle aspiration**). Direct smears of the fluid can be made, but most samples contain few cells.

Potential complications

- Catheter breakage and aspiration of the catheter into the airway
- Bronchospasm
- Laryngospasm and coughing
- Haemorrhage
- Iatrogenic infection
- Pneumothorax

Bronchoscopy

Indications/Use

- Evaluation of tracheal and lower airway disorders
- Acquisition of samples (see also **Bronchoalveolar lavage**)
- Foreign body removal

Contraindications

- Patient not stable enough to undergo anaesthesia (e.g. severe hypoxaemia, cardiac arrhythmia/dysfunction)
- Coagulopathy
- Partial tracheal obstruction
- Unstable asthma
- Pulmonary hypertension

Equipment

- Flexible endoscope: diameter 2.5–5 mm, length 25–80 cm
- Endoscopic viewing equipment
- Topical anaesthetic
- Mouth gag
- Elbow port: connects the endotracheal (ET) tube to the breathing circuit and allows simultaneous insertion of the endoscope whilst oxygen and the volatile agent are delivered
- Supplementary oxygen
- Pulse oximeter
- For foreign body retrieval: forceps including basket, rat-toothed, alligator, net and polyp snare-type

Patient preparation and positioning

- Inhalation anaesthesia is generally recommended, but if the patient is too small to have an endoscope passed through an ET tube, intravenous anaesthesia must be used. Intubation should only be performed if the endoscope can fit easily through the ET tube, allowing for movement of air and the endoscope at the same time. An elbow port connector should be used to provide constant gas anaesthesia whilst the endoscope is passed through the ET tube.
- Pre-oxygenation is very helpful, especially when there is compromised oxygenation. This can be provided through nasal oxygen delivery or a face mask. Supplementary oxygen can also

be delivered through the channel of the endoscope or via a catheter placed alongside the endoscope. Flow volumes of 1–3 litres per minute can be safely used.

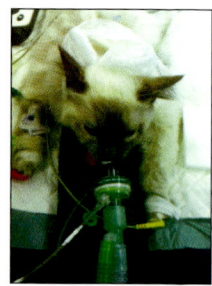

- Position the patient in sternal recumbency with the head elevated and neck extended.
- A mouth gag is essential to keep the mouth open and prevent the patient biting down on to the endoscope in the event of contact with the pharynx stimulating the gag reflex.

WARNINGS

- **Endoscopes should not remain in an airway for longer than 30–50 seconds, as they can interfere with ventilation and could result in hypercapnia and overventilation of the lungs, trauma and bronchospasm.**
- **If oxygen is being delivered through the channel constantly, carbon dioxide cannot escape through the same channel.**

SPECIAL CONSIDERATIONS FOR CATS

Extra care should be taken when performing bronchoscopy in cats, as their airways are particularly prone to bronchospasm.

- The procedure should be performed as quickly as possible, with the minimum of trauma.
- To reduce the risk of bronchospasm, terbutaline can be given approximately 30 minutes pre-bronchoscopy (0.015 mg/kg s.c. or i.m). Onset of action is 15–30 minutes and is usually notable by an increase in heart rate.
- Terbutaline should also be available for giving during the procedure if bronchospasm still occurs. If this does not stabilize the patient, consider administration of a short-acting steroid (e.g. dexamethasone sodium phosphate 0.1 mg/kg i.v. once).
- A suction unit (or 5 ml syringe attached to a sterile urinary catheter) should be kept nearby and can be used for clearing any secretions from the oropharynx. Try to maintain the cat in sternal recumbency. If the cat resents suctioning of the oropharynx, re-induction of anaesthesia may be required to clear the upper airway effectively.

Technique

1   Spray the larynx with topical anaesthetic to avoid laryngospasm.

2   Advance the endoscope into the larynx and examine this region.

3   If the patient is to be intubated, the proximal trachea should be evaluated prior to intubation. Intubation can be performed after evaluation of the length of the

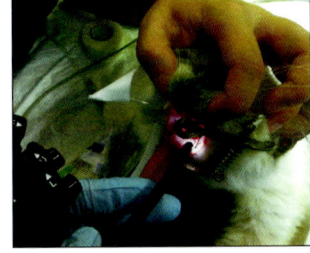

trachea that would otherwise be covered by the ET tube.

4   Centre the endoscope as it is advanced, and take care not to irritate the surface of the trachea with the endoscope.

5   As the endoscope is advanced, the carina or bifurcation is seen. The patient's right side is on the operator's left side; therefore, the right mainstem bronchus will be seen on the left side of the image. The left and right mainstem bronchi branch off crisply with sharp edges.

6   The right mainstem bronchus is in line with the trachea and should be examined first.

7   Then pass the endoscope into the left mainstem bronchus.

8   Evaluate segmental and subsegmental airways on the left and right sides as thoroughly and systematically as possible.

9   Take samples as required (see **Bronchoalveolar lavage**).

10 Following bronchoscopy, continue administration of 100% oxygen and volatile agent for 5 minutes, to allow time to detect any immediate complications of the procedure, e.g. bronchospasm. The animal's respiratory rate and pattern, and ideally pulse oximetry, should be monitored continuously during the procedure and in the recovery period following anaesthesia, due to the associated potential complications, which may induce dyspnoea and hypoxaemia.

11 Oxygen supplementation may need to be continued following extubation until the animal is able to maintain sternal recumbency and pulse oximetry shows adequate levels of oxygen saturation (S_pO_2 >95%). Respiratory pattern and rate should be monitored over the following 12 hours (in the hospital or by the owners if the animal recovers from the procedure without any immediate complications).

12 If complications occur in the recovery period and rapid reversal of hypoxaemia and dyspnoea cannot be achieved medically, re-induction of anaesthesia for intubation and ventilation may be required to increase oxygenation and enable investigations to determine the cause of dyspnoea.

Foreign body removal

1   Position the endoscope several centimetres proximal to the foreign body.

2   Pass the retrieval forceps, in the *closed* position, down the biopsy channel (if there is sufficient room) or adjacent to the endoscope.

3 Open the forceps, grasp the foreign body and close the forceps.
4 Remove the endoscope and forceps at the same time.

> **WARNINGS**
>
> - Care must be taken to provide adequate ventilation during the retrieval procedure.
> - Foreign body removal can be very challenging. The veterinary surgeon should be prepared to stop and refer the animal for surgery if the procedure becomes prolonged.
> - There is a risk of airway damage or rupture and the development of a pneumothorax. The equipment for thoracocentesis or thoracostomy tube placement should therefore be available.

Potential complications

- Bronchospasm
- Laryngospasm and coughing
- Haemorrhage
- Iatrogenic infection
- Pneumothorax

> **FURTHER INFORMATION**
>
> Further information on endoscopic equipment and techniques can be found in the *BSAVA Manual of Canine and Feline Endoscopy and Endosurgery*. Further information on bronchoscopy and its interpretation can be found in the *BSAVA Manual of Canine and Feline Cardiorespiratory Medicine*.

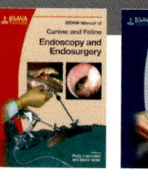
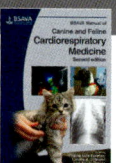

Buccal mucosal bleeding time

Indications/Use

- Suspected primary coagulopathy

Contraindications

- Thrombocytopenia
- Known primary haemostatic abnormality

Equipment

- Spring-loaded bleeding device (e.g. Surgicutt Vet H)
- 2 cm wide gauze bandage
- Tissue paper/filter paper
- Stopwatch or timer

Patient preparation and positioning

- If possible, the procedure should be performed with the animal conscious.
- Light sedation may be required in fractious dogs and in cats.
- The patient is restrained in lateral or sternal recumbency.

Technique

1 Fold back the patient's upper lip and hold it in place, either via an assistant or with a gauze bandage, in order to impede the venous return from the lip and cause congestion.

2 Position the bleeding device on the buccal mucosa, avoiding any obvious superficial vessels. Hold firmly but avoid excessive pressure.

3 Depress the trigger on the device to create a small incision in the buccal mucosa and simultaneously start the timer. Remove the bleeding device approximately 1 second after triggering.

4 At 15 seconds, blot the flow of blood with filter paper placed a few millimetres below the incision, without dislodging the clot.

5 Blot in a similar manner every 15 seconds until blood no longer stains the filter paper.

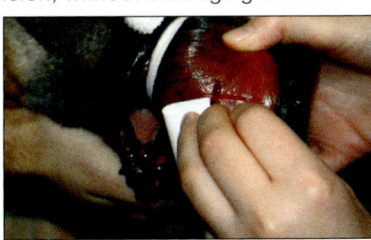

6 Stop the timer when bleeding has ceased.

7 Record the time from making the incision to cessation of bleeding.

Results

- In healthy dogs, BMBT is 1.7–3.3 minutes; this can be mildly prolonged (to 4.2 minutes) in anaesthetized or sedated dogs.
- BMBT of healthy anaesthetized cats is 1.0–2.4 minutes.
- Prolonged BMBT may indicate moderate to marked thrombocytopenia, thrombopathias (e.g. NSAID-induced), or von Willebrand's disease.

Potential complications

Prolonged bleeding can occur (uncommon) but should cease with continued pressure over the incision site. If it does not, the administration of fresh frozen plasma may be required.

FURTHER INFORMATION

Further details on coagulation tests and abnormalities can be found in the *BSAVA Manual of Canine and Feline Haematology and Transfusion Medicine.*

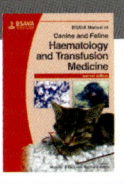

Cardiopulmonary resuscitation

Indications/Use

- Confirmed cardiopulmonary arrest (CPA) or in any unresponsive apnoeic cat or dog until CPA is ruled out

> **WARNINGS**
> - **Requires recognition of unresponsive apnoeic patient only, as basic CPR must not be delayed.**
> - ***Rapid*** **assessment of Airway, Breathing and Circulation required.**

Equipment

- Organized and regularly audited crash trolley, containing:
    - Cuffed endotracheal tubes (ET): full range of sizes with stylets and dog urinary catheters for difficult intubation
    - Ambu bag (self-re-inflating bag)
    - Intravenous catheters: range of sizes
    - Intraosseous catheters
    - Dog urinary catheters for intratracheal drug administration
    - Relevant drugs

Indication	Drug and concentration	Dose
Cardiac arrest	Adrenaline (1:1000; 1 mg/ml) – Low dose	0.01 mg/kg
	Adrenaline (1:1000; 1 mg/ml) –High dose	0.1 mg/kg
	Atropine (0.6 mg/ml)	0.04 mg/kg
Ventricular fibrillation or pulseless ventricular tachycardia	Lidocaine (20 mg/ml)	2 mg/kg
Drug reversal	Naloxone (0.4 mg/ml)	0.04 mg/kg
	Flumazenil (0.1 mg/ml)	0.01 mg/kg
	Atipamezole (5 mg/ml)	100 µg/kg

- Needles and syringes to match drug doses required
- Electrical defibrillator and paste/gel
- Bags of sterile fluids for intravenous administration: 0.9% saline and lactated Ringer's (Hartmann's) solution
- Intravenous fluid administration sets
- 0.9% saline to flush intravenous/intraosseous catheters

- ECG monitor, pads and gel
- ETCO$_2$ monitor (if possible)
- Oxygen saturation (S_pO_2) monitor
- Blood pressure monitor
- Thermometer
- Blood sample pots/tubes
- Charts (clear; in CPR area)
  - Local CPR protocol
  - Drug dosages – preferably in mg/kg and in ml for weights 5–50 kg
- Plastic trough positioning aids – range of sizes
- Oxygen supply with necessary tubing/breathing circuit

Patient preparation and positioning

- Lateral recumbency.

Technique

- **Priority is to begin basic life support.**
- **Start advanced life support and monitoring simultaneously if possible.**

TIPS FOR A SUCCESSFUL OUTCOME

- Well trained team with team leader
- Regular rehearsals
- The team leader must give clear orders, which are repeated back by the team member carrying out the task, to ensure the task is completed correctly

---

Basic life support (BLS)

NOTES

- Each BLS cycle lasts 2 minutes.
- Begin first cycle as soon as possible, and complete it uninterrupted.
- Chest compressions and ventilation are carried out simultaneously.
- Change person performing chest compressions between cycles to avoid fatigue.

Chest compressions

- **Perform 100–120 compressions per minute.**
- Compress the thorax by a third to a half of its resting width and allow full chest recoil between compressions.

Medium and large dogs: Place the palm of one hand over the back of the other hand with your fingers interdigitated. Apply the palms of the hands to the thorax of the animal. Keep your elbows locked in extension and push downwards through the palms of your hands. For most dogs, place hands centrally over the thorax such that compressive force acts on the widest part. Place hands directly over the heart for dogs with deep narrow chests.

Cats and small dogs: Wrap a single hand around the sternum at the level of the heart and compress the thorax between your thumb and fingers; or use the technique for deep narrow chested dogs.

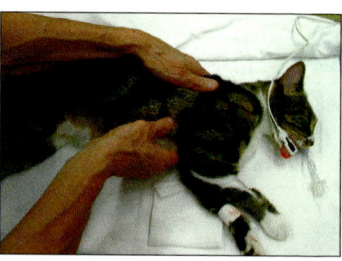

Ventilation

1 Endotracheal intubation of the animal in lateral recumbency.
2 Secure the ET tube to the animal's muzzle or mandible.
3 Inflate the cuff of the ET tube.
4 Attach an Ambu bag to the ET tube.
5 **Ventilate at 10 breaths/min with a tidal volume of 10 ml/kg and inspiratory time of 1 second.**

Monitoring

- **Electrocardiography** to look for arrhythmias.
- End-tidal CO_2 ($ETCO_2$): an indicator of correct placement of ET tube in trachea and adequacy of ventilation. Aim for $ETCO_2$ of >15 mmHg (dog) or >20 mmHg (cat).
- Pulse: palpate between BLS cycles; useful for detection of return of spontaneous circulation.
- Electrolytes and arterial blood gas: not mandatory but useful where electrolyte disturbance may be involved in causing CPA.

Advanced life support (ALS)

1 Establish vascular access: **intravenous catheter placement** (preferable) or **intraosseous cannula placement**.

> **NOTE**
>
> Intratracheal drug dosing can be considered for adrenaline (0.02–0.1 mg/kg) and atropine (0.15–0.2 mg/kg), but may be ineffective. Insert dog urinary catheter via ET tube to level of carina. Dilute drug with saline or sterile water.

2 Give low-dose adrenaline (0.01 mg/kg i.v.) during every other cycle of BLS. If CPA for >10 min, consider single high-dose adrenaline injection (0.1 mg/kg i.v.)
3 If asystole or pulseless electrical activity, give atropine (0.04 mg/kg iv) during every other cycle of BLS
4 If ventricular fibrillation (VF) or pulseless ventricular tachycardia (VT), perform **electrical defibrillation**:

- If VF or pulseless VT is detected within 4 minutes of CPA, perform defibrillation immediately
- If VF or pulseless VT is detected after 4 minutes of CPA, perform 1 cycle of BLS before defibrillation.

i   To avoid the risk of fire, make sure there is no alcohol on the fur of the thorax.
ii Set the electrical dose.

Monophasic defibrillation	
External	4–6 J/kg
Internal	0.5–1 J/kg

iii Apply defibrillator gel or paste to the paddles.
iv   Press the paddles firmly against opposite sides of the thorax, over the heart, at the level of the costochondral junctions.
v   If two hand paddles are used, the animal will need to be placed in dorsal recumbency; a plastic trough positioning aid will help.
vi   If a posterior paddle is available, the animal can remain in lateral recumbency. The posterior paddle is positioned between the table and the animal, and the hand paddle is placed on the opposite side of the thorax.
vii Charge the defibrillator.
viii Operator calls 'Clear!' and ensures that no-one (including themselves) is touching the patient or table.
ix   Current is applied to the thorax.
x   Perform 1 cycle of BLS.
xi   Reassess ECG.
xii If VF or pulseless VT, repeat electrical defibrillation with a 50% increased dose.

> **NOTE**
>
> If electrical defibrillation is unavailable, give 2 mg/kg i.v. bolus of lidocaine, but this may be ineffective.

5 Administer reversal agents for opioids (naloxone), alpha-2 agonists (atipamezole) or benzodiazepines (flumazenil), if these drugs are implicated in CPA (see table for doses).
6 Supplement inspired oxygen.
- If arterial blood gas data are available, titrate to P_aO_2 of 80–105 mmHg.
- If arterial blood gas data are unavailable, giving 100% of F_iO_2 is reasonable.
7 Consider intravenous fluid therapy.
- In euvolaemic or hypervolaemic patient, do not give fluids.
- In hypovolaemic patient, give intravenous fluids to restore blood volume, but cautiously (1–2 ml/kg/h).

8   Open-chest CPR. *Only consider this if a specialist veterinary team and a dedicated intensive care unit are available.*

Summary

> **Basic life support (BLS)**
>
> Perform in uninterrupted cycles of 2 minutes each:
> - Chest compressions: 100–120/min; compress thorax width by one-third to one-half
> - Intubate and ventilate: 10 breaths/min; tidal volume 10 ml/kg; inspiratory time 1 second

> **Monitoring**
>
> - ECG to check for arrhythmias
> - End-tidal CO_2: aim with good chest compressions: Dog >15 mmHg; Cat >20 mmHg
> - Palpate pulse between BLS cycles

> **Obtain vascular access**

> **Treat arrhythmias**
>
> - Asystole or pulseless electrical activity:
>   - Give low-dose adrenaline every other BLS cycle
>   - Give atropine every other BLS cycle
>   - *If no response after 10 minutes*, give high-dose adrenaline
> - Ventricular fibrillation or pulseless ventricular tachycardia:
>   - Electrical defibrillation
>   - *If no response after 1 BLS cycle consider:* lidocaine, low-dose adrenaline every other BLS cycle, or electrical defibrillation with a 50% increased dose

> **Administer reversal agents**
>
> - For opioids: Naloxone
> - For alpha-2 agonists: Atipamezole
> - For benzodiazepines: Flumazenil

> **Supplement oxygen**
>
> - Give F_iO_2 of 100%, or titrate to P_aO_2 of 80–105 mmHg

Post-CPR care

- Referral to a specialist centre should be considered.
- Continue monitoring: ECG; $ETCO_2$; S_pO_2; arterial blood gases; blood pressure; blood electrolyte, lactate and glucose concentrations; and body temperature.
- Assess for return of spontaneous respiration. Normal respiratory function is associated with:
  - $ETCO_2$ 27–38 mmHg (dog) or 21–31 mmHg (cat)
  - P_aCO_2 32–43 mmHg (dog) or 26–36 mmHg
  - S_pO_2 94–98%
  - P_aO_2 80–100 mmHg.
- If hypoxaemic or hyperoxaemic, change the amount of supplemental oxygen appropriately.
- Intermittent positive pressure ventilation (IPPV) will be required if P_aCO_2 is abnormal, or animal is hypoxaemic despite F_iO_2 of 60%.
- Assess haemodynamic status. A normal haemodynamic status is associated with:
  - Mean arterial pressure 80–120 mmHg
  - Systolic arterial pressure 100–200 mmHg.
- If hypertensive, decrease any vasopressor treatment; treat pain; and consider antihypertensives, *but hypertension may be advantageous immediately post CPR.*
- If hypotensive, consider: fluid therapy if hypovolaemic; vasopressors if vasodilated; inotropes if decreased heart contractility; blood transfusion if anaemic.
- If normotensive but lactate >2.5 mmol/l, consider treatment for poor perfusion and follow guidelines above for hypotension.
- Assess temperature.
  - Mild hypothermia (32–34°C) may be advantageous during CPA.
  - Hypothermic animals should be rewarmed slowly – by 0.25–0.5°C per hour.
- Assess neurological status:
  - Assess for signs of cerebral oedema: coma, cranial nerve deficits, decerebrate postures, abnormal mentation. If cerebral oedema suspected, consider treatment with mannitol or hypertonic saline.
  - Assess for signs of seizures, though seizure activity may be undetectable. Overt seizures should be treated: see **Seizures – emergency protocol**. Prophylaxis with phenobarbital loading may be considered in an apparently normal patient.

FURTHER INFORMATION

Further information on CPR is available in the *BSAVA Manual of Canine and Feline Emergency and Critical Care* (new edition due 2015). See also Fletcher *et al.* (2012) RECOVER evidence and knowledge gap analysis on veterinary CPR. Part 7: Clinical guidelines. *J Vet Emerg Crit Care* **22**(S1), 102–131.

Cast application

Indications/Use

- Additional external support to supplement internal fixation for:
    - Arthrodesis of carpus/tarsus
    - Fractures of the distal limb
- Primary coaptation of *selected* long bone fractures that meet the following criteria:
    - Fractures *distal to the elbow and stifle*
    - *Relatively stable fracture configuration*, e.g. greenstick fractures, interdigitating transverse fractures, or fracture of one member of a pair of bones
    - Minimally displaced fractures with at least *50% overlap of the fracture ends in orthogonal radiographic views*
    - *Non-articular* fractures
    - *A predicted fracture union time of 4–6 weeks, as assessed by radiography; juvenile animals are better candidates than adults.*

Contraindications

- Soft tissue swelling
- Primary coaptation of fractures that do not fit the above criteria, including unstable spiral and oblique fractures, all comminuted fractures and all articular fractures
- Primary coaptation of fractures of the distal radius and ulna in small breed dogs
- Athletic or working animals

> **NOTES**
> - Effective cast application is challenging in obese animals and chondrodystrophoid breeds
> - Sight hounds have a higher incidence of cast complications

Equipment

- Non-adhesive dressing for any wounds
- Adhesive tape for stirrups (2.5 cm wide)
- Tongue depressor
- Stockinette (not absolutely essential)
- 2 to 3 rolls of cast padding (5–7.5 cm wide)
- 2 to 3 rolls of conforming gauze bandage (5–7.5 cm wide)
- 2 to 3 rolls of resin-impregnated fibreglass cast materials
- Outer protective bandage material, e.g. self-adhesive non-adherent bandage or adhesive bandage (optional)

Patient preparation and positioning

- The animal should be sedated heavily or anaesthetized.
- The haircoat should be clipped if it is likely to interfere with cast application, and the limb should be clean and dry.

- The animal should be placed in lateral recumbency with the affected limb uppermost and supported in a weight-bearing position by an assistant.

Technique

1 Place two strips of adhesive tape (stirrups) on the distal limb on *either* the dorsal and palmar/plantar surfaces, *or* the medial and lateral surfaces. These stirrups should extend beyond the tip of the toes and should be stuck to each other or to a tongue depressor. The assistant can now maintain the limb elevated away from the body by holding the stirrups.

2 Roll the stockinette up the limb and apply tension to eliminate creases. (*optional*)

3 Beginning distally, apply cast padding in a spiral fashion up the limb, overlapping by 50% on each turn. Two layers are generally indicated. Take particular care to ensure even padding over pressure points. Excessive padding about pressure points should be avoided, and consideration should be given to increasing the padding in adjacent depressed regions to create a bandage of even diameter.

4 Apply conforming gauze to compact the cast padding, again overlapping turns by 50%.

5 Follow the manufacturers' recommendations regarding wetting and handling of the cast material.

6 Apply the cast material over the bandage, again with a 50% overlap on each turn. Two (cats and most dogs) or three (for large dogs or giant breeds) layers of cast material should be applied. Leave a 1–2 cm margin of cast padding exposed proximal to the cast. Increase tension as the cast is applied proximal to the elbow or stifle, to give a snug fit about the muscle masses and to prevent loosening. Do not make indentations in the cast material with fingers.

7 Once the cast has hardened, an oscillating saw may be used to trim excess casting material proximally and distally to prevent rubbing and to permit weight bearing, respectively.

8 Split the cast into halves along either the sagittal or frontal planes using an oscillating saw: the plane chosen should result in least compromise to supportive function of the cast, as determined by fracture configuration and forces acting on the cast. Hold the cast together with adhesive tape. *Splitting the cast in half simplifies and facilitates cast changes, encouraging regular checking of the limb for healing and complications.*

9 Roll the stockinette and padding over the proximal edge of the cast and secure them to the cast with adhesive tape.

10 Peel apart the stirrups, twist them through 180 degrees and stick them to the distal cast. The pads and nails of the axial digits should remain exposed.

11 Medication with non-steroidal anti-inflammatory drugs is useful to limit soft tissue swelling and to provide analgesia. The requirement for ongoing treatment should be reassessed after 3–5 days.

Cast maintenance and monitoring

- Written instructions should always be given out at discharge and owners must understand their role in cast maintenance.
- Casts should be checked every 4 hours for the first 24 hours and then weekly by a veterinary surgeon; rapidly growing dogs and other high-risk patients may require more frequent assessment.
- Animals with a cast should have restricted exercise levels.
- The cast must be kept clean and dry. A plastic bag may be placed over the foot while the dog is walking outside. The plastic bag should be removed when the dog is indoors.

CHECKING PROCEDURE

- Splitting the cast in half simplifies and facilitates cast changes, encouraging regular checking of the limb for healing and complications.
  1. Remove the adhesive tape securing the two halves of the cast and remove the cast.
  2. Remove conforming gauze and cast padding.
  3. Remove dressing if present.
  4. Examine any wounds and the limb for cast complications.
  5. Reapply dressing as required.
  6. Reapply cast padding and gauze padding, taking care to use the same amount as before to prevent undue pressure or looseness.
  7. Reapply both halves of the cast and secure with adhesive tape.

- Points to monitor for are:
  - Swelling of the toes or proximal limb
  - Toe discoloration and coolness
  - Skin abrasion about the toes or proximal cast
  - Cast loosening
  - Angular deformity
  - Cast damage or breakage
  - Discharge or foul odour
  - Chewing at the cast
  - Deterioration in weight-bearing function
  - Signs of general ill health (inappetence, dullness, etc.).

These signs should prompt cast removal, assessment and replacement only if appropriate.

Potential complications

- Venous stasis
- Limb oedema
- Moist dermatitis
- Skin maceration under a wet bandage
- Infection

- Pressure sores/skin necrosis
- Cast loosening
- Deterioration in fracture apposition
- Fracture non-union, malunion or delayed union
- Joint stiffness or laxity

Cast removal and aftercare

- The timing of cast removal should be aided by radiography. In most instances radiographic evidence of bridging callus formation across fracture sites or arthrodesis sites is desired prior to cast removal.
- After cast removal it is important that a regimen of progressively increasing controlled exercise is enforced. The goal is stimulation of callus remodelling without jeopardizing fracture/arthrodesis repair.

Cerebrospinal fluid sampling

Indications

- Suspected meningitis
- Infectious or inflammatory CNS disease
- Pyrexia of unknown origin
- Suspected CNS lymphoma

SITE SELECTION

- CSF is more commonly collected from the **cerebellomedullary cistern** as it is easier, usually results in a larger sample volume, and is typically associated with less iatrogenic blood contamination than collection from the lumbar cistern.
- In cases of focal CNS disease, samples are more likely to be abnormal when they are collected caudal to the lesion. Therefore, in animals with lesions involving the spinal cord or canal, **lumbar cistern** samples are more consistently abnormal than samples collected from the cerebellomedullary cistern.
- Collection from both sites can be considered in cases of diffuse pathology or when one of the samples is contaminated.

(a) Cerebellomedullary cistern

Contraindications

- Signs suggestive of raised intracranial pressure (e.g. progressive obtundation; initial miosis then later fixed mydriasis; extensor rigidity; opisthotonos; irregular respiration)

- Evidence of a large intracranial space-occupying mass on CT/MRI
- Evidence of severe hydrocephalus or severe cerebral oedema on CT/MRI
- Evidence of brain herniation on CT/MRI
- Suspected active intracranial haemorrhage or haemorrhagic diathesis
- Atlantoaxial luxation or other causes of cervical vertebral instability
- Infection of the soft tissues overlying the puncture site
- Patient with a high risk of anaesthetic complications

> **WARNING**
>
> - Caution should be employed with Cavalier King Charles Spaniels. Numbers of this breed are affected with Chiari-like malformations, and sampling from the cerebellomedullary cistern may lead to needle penetration of the cerebellum and brainstem. It is therefore advisable to obtain a lumbar cistern sample unless there is MRI evidence to show that the cerebellum is not caudally displaced.

Equipment

- As required for **Aseptic preparation – (b) non-surgical procedures**
- Spinal needle:
    - 20 G (large dogs) to 22 G (cats and small dogs)
    - 1.5 inches (most dogs and cats) to 3.0 inches (some large dogs or giant dog breeds)
- Sterile gloves
- EDTA and sterile plain collection tubes
- Sedimentation chamber

Patient preparation and positioning

- General anaesthesia is essential.
- The animal is placed in lateral recumbency, with the dorsum near the edge of the table.
- Flex the head to 90 degrees and have an assistant hold it in place.

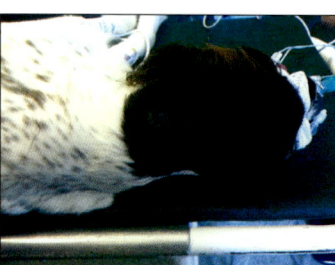 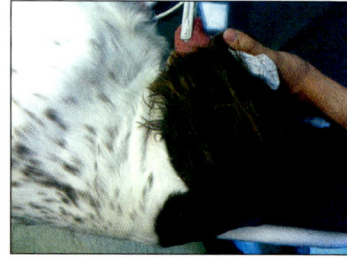

WARNING
■ **Flexing the neck may compromise respiration. Monitor the animal's respiratory rate and character at all times. Ideally, an armoured endotracheal (ET) tube should be placed. If not, then silicone tubes are preferable to rubber ones as the latter may kink and obstruct the airways.**

■ Raise the muzzle until its sagittal plane is parallel with the table top.

■ **Aseptic preparation – (a) non-surgical procedures** is performed on a wide area at the base of the skull, from the occipital protuberance to the crest of the axis, including the wings of the atlas.

■ It is advisable to wear sterile gloves to reduce the likelihood of introducing infection during the procedure.

Technique

1 Palpate a triangle of landmarks formed by the occipital protuberance and the most prominent points of the lateral wings of the atlas.

2 The location for needle insertion is on the dorsal midline. It can be visualized as being at the centre of a triangle formed by the occipital protuberance and the most prominent points of the lateral wings of the atlas.

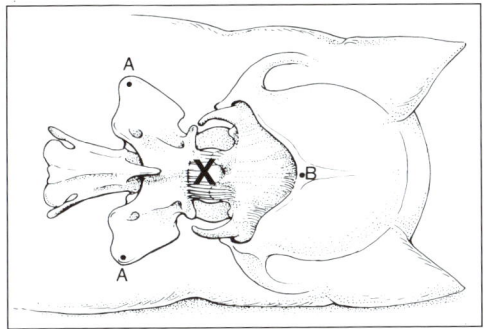

Needle insertion site (X). A = atlas. B = occipital protuberance

Alternatively, the occipital protuberance can be used to identify the midline, and the needle inserted just cranial to the most cranial aspect of the wings of the atlas.

3 Insert the spinal needle parallel to the table surface in the direction of the muzzle, with the bevel facing caudally.

4 Once the skin is penetrated, remove the stylet.

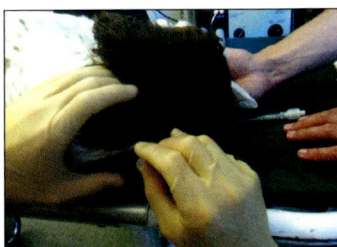

5 Advance the needle very slowly (1–2 mm at a time) whilst watching for CSF to appear in the hub. If the needle hits bone while being advanced, it may be redirected cranially or caudally, moving the needle off the bone until the subarachnoid space is penetrated. If this is not successful after a

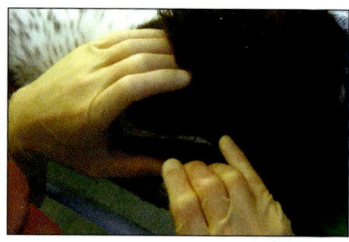

few redirections, remove the needle and try again.

6 A characteristic 'pop' might be felt when the needle passes through the atlanto-occipital membrane. When the subarachnoid space has been entered, CSF will appear in the needle hub. If blood is seen in the needle hub, entry into a local blood vessel is likely and the sample will be less useful for cytological evaluation. Remove the needle and make a fresh attempt with a new needle.

7 Collect CSF by allowing it to drip passively from the hub into collecting vessels. Suction with a syringe should *not* be applied.

8 When a minimum of 0.5 ml of CSF has been collected, withdraw the needle in a single motion.

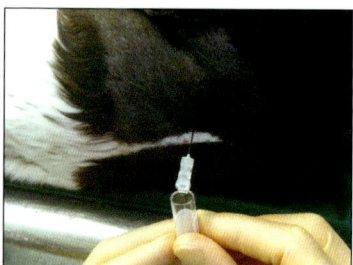

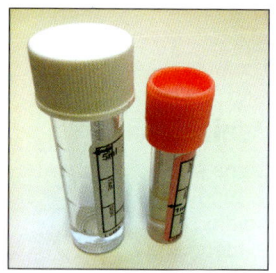

Sample handling

- CSF is hypotonic compared to serum; the cells within CSF swell rapidly and burst due to osmotic lysis soon after collection. Ideally, CSF should be either analysed or preserved for analysis within 30–60 minutes of collection.

- Most CSF samples contain relatively few cells; therefore, the sample can be concentrated by some means prior to microscopic examination. Cells can be concentrated using a homemade sedimentation chamber. The flanged end of a 2 ml syringe barrel (the end where the plunger would be inserted) is clamped to a clean microscope slide using bulldog clips after smearing Vaseline or another occlusive lubricant around the base to form an airtight seal. 0.25–0.5 ml of CSF is put into the chamber and left for 30 minutes; the supernatant is then removed using a pipette. The slide with adherent cells is then air-dried and submitted to the laboratory unstained. Other tests can be performed on the supernatant.

- *Alternatively,* rather than concentrating the cells, they can be preserved by the addition of 30–50% by volume of the animal's own serum (i.e. 0.3–0.5 ml serum to 1.0 ml CSF). This will preserve the CSF cells for up to 48 hours after collection. **If this is done, it is important also to submit a CSF sample in a plain tube without the addition of serum to enable total protein measurement and any other analyses.**

■ CSF in an EDTA tube is submitted for cytological examination, total protein and total nucleated cell count.
■ CSF in an EDTA tube can also be submitted for the detection of infectious diseases by PCR.
■ CSF in a sterile plain tube can be submitted for serology, bacteriological or fungal culture if required.

Potential complications

■ Cerebral and/or cerebellar herniation due to changes in intracranial pressure, resulting in brainstem signs, respiratory arrest and death
■ Brainstem trauma due to needle puncture
■ CNS haemorrhage
■ Loss of airway patency due to patient positioning and use of an unarmoured ET tube
■ Iatrogenic infection

(b) Lumbar cistern

Contraindications

■ Signs suggestive of raised intracranial pressure (e.g. progressive obtundation; initial miosis than later fixed mydriasis; extensor rigidity; opisthotonos; irregular respiration)
■ Evidence of brain herniation on CT/MRI
■ Suspected active intracranial haemorrhage or haemorrhagic diathesis
■ Luxation or vertebral instability of the caudal lumbar vertebrae
■ Empyema or spinal epidural abscess
■ Infection of the soft tissues overlying the puncture site
■ Patient at high risk of anaesthetic complications

Equipment

■ As required for collection from the **cerebellomedullary cistern**
■ Spinal needle:
  ▪ 20 G (large or giant dog breeds) to 22 G (cats and small dogs)
  ▪ 1.5 inches (cats) to 2–3 inches (dogs)

Patient preparation and positioning

■ General anaesthesia is essential.
■ The animal is placed in lateral recumbency, with its dorsum near the edge of the table.

- Flex the lumbar spine by moving the hindlimbs cranially and have an assistant hold the animal in this position.
- Locate the appropriate intervertebral space:
    - Dogs: L4–L5 or, preferably, L5–L6
    - Cats: L5–L6 or, potentially, L6–L7

  This is done by palpating the iliac crests: the small, difficult-to-palpate vertebral spinous process found between the iliac crests is L7; the much more prominent vertebral spinous process immediately cranial to the iliac crests is that of L6.
- **Aseptic preparation – (a) non-surgical procedures** is performed over an area at least 5 cm wide.

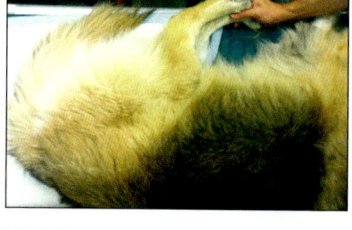

Technique

1   The needle is inserted at an angle of 45 degrees to the skin, on the midline, and just caudal to the appropriate vertebral spinous process (e.g. caudal to the spinous process of L6 to reach the L5/L6 space), with the bevel facing cranially.

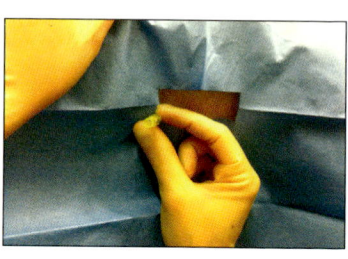

2   Once the skin is penetrated, advance the needle until it hits bone (the dorsal lamina). The stylet may be left within the spinal needle.

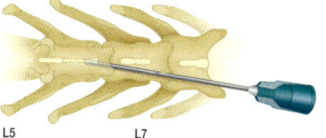

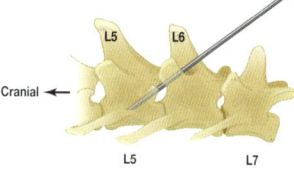

3   'Walking' the needle over the dorsal lamina is often required to arrive at the resistant interarcuate ligament. Allow the needle to pass through the interarcuate ligament.

4   When the needle passes through the cauda equina/caudal spinal cord, this often elicits a tail or leg twitch.

5   The needle is advanced to the bottom of the spinal canal. Remove the stylet and wait for CSF to flow.

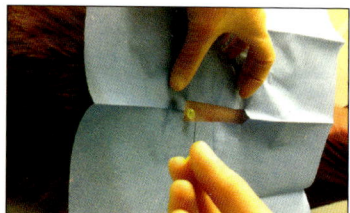

6 When the subarachnoid space has been entered, CSF will appear in the needle hub. If no CSF appears, retract the needle slightly or turn the hub gently. If blood emerges from the needle hub, entry into a local blood vessel is likely and the sample will be less useful for cytological evaluation. Remove the needle and make a fresh attempt with a new needle.

7 Collect CSF by allowing it to drip passively from the hub into collecting vessels. Suction with a syringe should *not* be applied.

8 When a minimum of 0.5 ml CSF has been collected, withdraw the needle in a single motion.

9 Fluoroscopic/radiographic needle guidance might be helpful in some cases.

Sample handling

As for **(a) cerebellomedullary cistern**.

Potential complications

- Cerebral and/or cerebellar herniation due to changes in intracranial pressure resulting in brainstem signs, respiratory arrest and death
- Spinal cord trauma due to needle puncture
- CNS haemorrhage
- Iatrogenic infection

Cystocentesis

Indications/Use

- Collection of urine directly from the bladder without contamination from the urethra or genital tract, e.g. for bacterial culture
- Decompression of a severely overdistended bladder pending urethral catheterization or, in exceptional circumstances, when urethral catheterization is not possible

Contraindications

- Severely diseased bladder (rupture possible)
- Inadequate bladder volume or excessive body fat such that the bladder cannot be palpated or immobilized manually
- Potential pyometra or prostatic abscess that could be inadvertently ruptured by this technique
- Bladder tumour that could potentially be seeded

Equipment

- As required for **Aseptic preparation – (a) non-surgical procedures**
- Hypodermic needles:
  - Dogs: 21–23 G, 1–2 inches
  - Cats: 23 G, 1–2 inches
- 10 ml syringe
- Two sterile plain collection tubes capable of holding at least 5 ml each

> ## BACTERIOLOGY
>
> - If bacteriology is to be performed at an external laboratory, urine should be placed in a sterile plain collection tube and be analysed within 24 hours of collection.
> - Note that the use of a container containing boric acid preservative (red top universal container) is no longer recommended.

Patient preparation and positioning

- Cystocentesis can usually be performed with the patient under physical restraint or light sedation.
- It can be performed with the animal in either dorsal or lateral recumbency, or with the animal standing.
- *Alternatively*, cystocentesis can be perfomed under ultrasound guidance.
- **Aseptic preparation – (a) non-surgical procedures** is performed over the appropriate area.

Technique

With the animal in dorsal or lateral recumbency:

1. With one hand palpate and stabilize the bladder by pushing it in a caudal direction against the pelvic brim.
2. Attach the needle to the syringe and insert through the abdominal wall, on the midline, just in front of the pelvic brim.

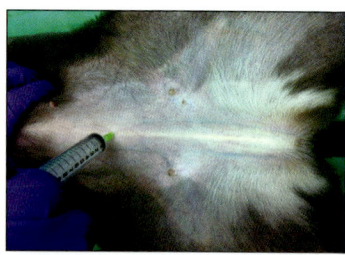

In the standing animal, urine should ideally be obtained from the right side (to avoid penetrating the descending colon), while gently pushing the bladder from the left side towards the right side of the caudal abdomen. Alternatively, a left-sided approach can be used, with the bladder gently pushed from the right side toward the left.

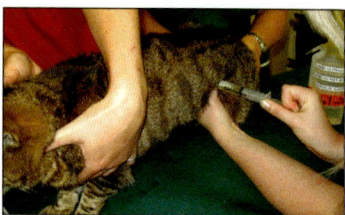

From *BSAVA Manual of Feline Practice* and courtesy of Langford Veterinary Services

3. The ideal site of bladder penetration is a short distance (a few centimetres, but will depend on the degree of bladder fill) cranial to the junction of the bladder and the urethra. If possible, insert

the needle in a caudal direction, at a 45-degree angle to the bladder wall (so that the layers of the bladder wall will help to seal the puncture site).

4   Apply slight negative pressure to the syringe while inserting the needle.

5   Once the bladder lumen is penetrated, urine will be seen filling the syringe. Continue to stabilize the bladder until you withdraw the needle from the abdomen.

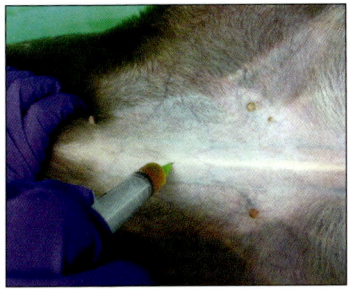

6   Once sufficient urine is collected to perform the required diagnostic tests (usually a minimum of 5 ml), remove the needle in one motion.

Sample handling

- Urine should be placed into a sterile plain tube for bacterial culture and should reach the laboratory as soon as possible, within 24 hours.
- A separate sample in a plain tube can be used for **Urinalysis**.

Potential complications

- Very rarely, an overdistended and traumatized bladder will rupture during cystocentesis. Surgical repair is then required
- Uroperitoneum, following urine leaking from the needle site

Dexamethasone suppression test – low dose

Indications/use

- Aid to the diagnosis of canine hyperadrenocorticism (HAC): reliably identifies the majority of adrenal-dependent cases and 90–95% of dogs with pituitary-dependent HAC
- Aid to the diagnosis of feline HAC: reliably identifies the majority of adrenal- and pituitary-dependent cases

Equipment

- As for **Blood sampling – (b) venous**
- Dexamethasone suitable for intravenous administration
- Hypodermic needles: 21 G; ¾ to 1 inch
- Intravenous catheter
- 1 ml syringe
- Heparin or plain tubes

Patient preparation and positioning

- This procedure should be carried out in the conscious animal, using manual restraint.
- Positioning and skin preparation are as for **Blood sampling – (b) venous**.
- Ideally, the patient should be hospitalized for the duration of the test; avoid excessive exercise or stress.
- Alternatively, for patients that become stressed during hospitalization, they can be sent home between blood collection times. When at home they should be kept quiet, and not exercised or fed.

Technique

1 Collect a blood sample (approximately 2 ml) from the *jugular vein* and place it into a heparin or plain collection tube to enable measurement of the basal cortisol concentration.

2 Inject **0.01 mg/kg** (dogs) or **0.1 mg/kg** (cats) of dexamethasone into the *cephalic vein*.

> **NOTE**
>
> When dealing with a very small dose of dexamethasone, it is preferable to place an **intravenous catheter** to ensure that the entire dose is administered.

3 After 3 hours, collect a blood sample (approximately 2 ml) from the *jugular vein* and place into a heparin or plain tube. Label the tube clearly as the +3 hours sample.

4 After 8 hours, collect a further blood sample (approximately 2 ml) from the *jugular vein* and place into a heparin or plain tube. Label the tube clearly as the +8 hours sample.

5 Separate the serum or plasma prior to sending the samples to the laboratory.

FURTHER INFORMATION

For interpretation of results see the *BSAVA Manual of Canine and Feline Endocrinology*.

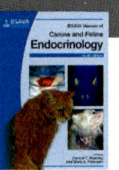

Diagnostic peritoneal lavage

Indications/Use

- The presence of a small volume of abdominal effusion that cannot be sampled by abdominocentesis, even under ultrasound guidance
- Where there is a suspicion of abdominal disease but no peritoneal fluid is visible, even with ultrasonography

---

NOTE

Diagnostic peritoneal lavage (DPL) should only be performed *after* four-quadrant **abdominocentesis** or ultrasound-guided aspiration

---

Contraindications

- Coagulopathy
- Marked distension of an abdominal viscus
- Marked organomegaly

Equipment

- As required for **Aseptic preparation – (a) non-surgical procedures**
- A large-bore 10–14 G over-the-needle catheter. The cannula can be fenestrated whilst on the metal stylet:
  - Use V-shaped incisions to create 2 or 3 fenestrations in a spiral pattern around the catheter
  - Do not make fenestrations directly opposite each other, as this would weaken the catheter

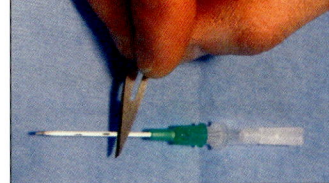

- Holes should not extend beyond 50% of the circumference of the catheter, to avoid risk of breakage
- No burrs must remain, as this could impair entry and exit of the catheter

- Local anaesthetic solution
- No. 11 or 15 scalpel
- 500 ml pre-warmed (to approximately 37°C) 0.9% sterile saline or lactated Ringer's solution (Hartmann's)
- Extension tubing
- 3-way tap
- 60 ml syringes
- 2 ml syringe
- EDTA and sterile plain collection tubes
- Microscope slides

Patient preparation and positioning

- Depending on the temperament of the patient, sedation may be required in order to minimize movement and avoid accidental puncture of abdominal organs.
- The patient is restrained in lateral recumbency.
- **Aseptic preparation – (a) non-surgical procedures** is carried out on an area approximately 10 cm x 10 cm, centred on the umbilicus, and a fenestrated drape placed.

Technique

1 The site for diagnostic peritoneal lavage is a point approximately 1–2 cm caudal to the umbilicus and 1 cm below the midline.

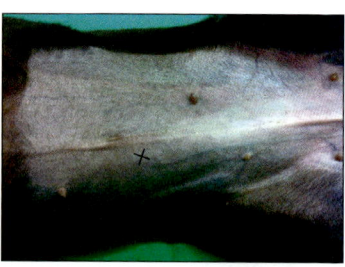

2 The skin and subcutaneous tissue may be infiltrated with local anaesthetic, if required.
3 Using a scalpel, make a 1–2 mm stab incision through the skin.
4 Introduce the fenestrated catheter and aim it caudally towards the pelvis. Once the abdominal wall is penetrated, remove the stylet, leaving the cannula in place.
5 Attach a 2 ml syringe and gently aspirate. **If sufficient fluid is obtained, diagnostic peritoneal lavage is not required.**
6 If no or insufficient fluid is obtained, attach a 3-way tap and extension tubing.
7 Infuse warm saline into the abdomen via gravity flow or gentle injection. A total volume of 20 ml/kg bodyweight is infused over approximately 5 minutes.
8 Gently roll the animal from side to side to distribute the fluid, preferably with the catheter still *in situ.*

9 Remove the 3-way tap and allow the fluid to drain into the collection tubes.

10 If no fluid is obtained, attempt gentle aspiration with a 2 ml syringe. **NB** Only a very small portion of the infused volume will be retrieved (usually only 1–2 ml); any remaining fluid will be absorbed across the peritoneal membrane.

Sample handling

- Place fluid in an EDTA tube for cytology. Note that a total nucleated cell count can *not* be performed, as the dilution factor is unknown.
- Place fluid in a plain tube for total protein measurement and other biochemical/serological tests.
- A sample in a sterile plain tube can be submitted for bacteriological culture if necessary.
- Make several fresh air-dried smears (unstained).

Potential complications

- **If blood is aspirated, stop.** Place the blood in a glass tube and observe for clot formation (see **Whole blood clotting time**). Blood from the abdominal cavity will not clot, whereas blood from a vessel or organ *will* clot. If bleeding persists, abdominal pressure should be applied via manual compression or a pressure bandage. Exploratory surgery may be required if bleeding persists and results in significant blood loss
- If fluid is obtained, suggesting puncture of the gastrointestinal tract, any hole should seal when the needle is removed. The patient should, however, be monitored for developing peritonitis
- In some animals with large abdominal effusions, the centesis hole may continue to drain fluid. If this occurs, a pressure dressing should be applied for several hours
- Extension of localized peritonitis
- Dissemination of neoplastic cells

FURTHER INFORMATION

Details of the cytological evaluation of peritoneal fluid samples are given in the *BSAVA Manual of Canine and Feline Clinical Pathology.*

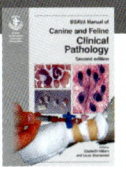

Edrophonium response test

Indications/Use

- Aid to the diagnosis of myasthenia gravis (MG) in dogs and cats (previously known as the Tensilon test). Note that not all animals with MG show a positive response to the test, and some animals with other forms of neuromuscular weakness will also show improvement. The test is more useful for generalized than for focal forms of MG

Contraindications

- Bronchial disease, especially feline asthma
- Bradycardia or other arrhythmias
- Mechanical gastrointestinal or urinary tract obstruction
- Hypotension
- Epilepsy

Equipment

- Edrophonium for intravenous injection
- Intravenous catheter
- Hypodermic needles: 21 G; ¾ to 1 inch
- 1 ml syringes
- Sterile 0.9% saline in a 5 ml syringe
- Atropine

Patient preparation and positioning

- This procedure should be carried out in the conscious animal.
- Skin preparation is as for **Intravenous catheter placement – (a) peripheral veins**.
- Place a catheter into a peripheral vein.
- The animal should then be exercised to induce muscle weakness (if appropriate).

Technique

1 Inject **0.1 mg/kg** (dogs; maximum dose 5 mg) or **0.25 mg/cat** of edrophonium *into the peripheral vein via the catheter*.

2 In a positive test, improvement in muscle strength should be noted within 30 seconds, with the effects dissipating within 5 minutes.

3 If there is no response, repeat the test after 10–20 minutes using **0.2 mg/kg** (dogs; maximum dose 5 mg) or **0.5 mg/cat** of edrophonium.

> **WARNING**
>
> - Atropine should be available (0.05 mg/kg i.v.) to control cholinergic side effects, e.g. aggravation of weakness, tremors, salivation, bradycardia, miosis, dyspnoea, urination, vomiting, diarrhoea.

Potential complications

- Cholinergic side effects (see above)

Ehmer sling

Indications/Use

- To support the hip joint following closed reduction of craniodorsal hip joint luxation (to permit stabilization and healing of the periarticular tissues)
- The Ehmer sling holds the pelvic limb in flexion, while internally rotating and mildly abducting the hip joint

Contraindications

- Hip instability following closed reduction of hip luxation, such that the Ehmer sling would not hold the hip in the reduced position: if the hip reluxates immediately after reduction or within 4 weeks, consider internal reduction and stabilization
- Ventral hip luxation
- Patient's temperament will not tolerate prolonged immobilization of limb
- Patient's conformation (e.g. chondrodystrophoid, well muscled) does not permit effective sling application
- Concurrent hip fractures or pre-existing disease (e.g. hip dysplasia)
- Concurrent injuries such as fractures or open wounds

Equipment

- Padded bandage material or cast padding
- Conforming gauze bandage
- Adhesive outer protective bandage material (e.g. Elastoplast)

Patient preparation and positioning

- General anaesthesia is required for closed reduction of hip luxation and is preferred for Ehmer sling application.
- The patient should be positioned in lateral recumbency with the affected limb uppermost.
- At the beginning of the procedure the pelvic limb should be held in a gently flexed position.

Technique

1   Confirm successful hip joint reduction by radiography and check range of motion and stability of the hip joint. Confirm that conservative management of hip luxation is appropriate (see **Hip luxation – closed reduction**).

2   Apply padded bandage material around the metatarsal region to lightly pad this area.

3   Secure the padded bandage material around the metatarsal region with conforming gauze bandage. It is important to pass the conforming gauze bandage from lateral to medial around the *dorsal* aspect of the metatarsus and from medial to lateral around the *plantar* aspect of the metatarsus.

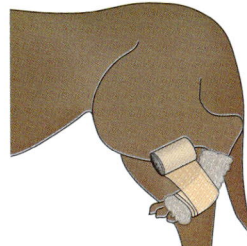

4 Completely flex the whole limb.
5 Pass the conforming gauze bandage from the *lateral* aspect of the metatarsus across the *cranial* aspect of the mid-tibia, to the *medial* aspects of the mid-tibia and mid-femur.

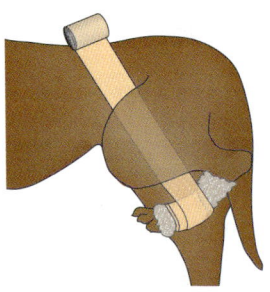

6 Pass the bandage over the *cranial* aspect of the mid-femur to the *lateral* aspect of the mid-femur.
7 Pass the bandage *caudal* to the stifle to the *medial* aspects of distal tibia and proximal metatarsal region, before returning to the *plantar* aspect of the metatarsus.
8 The result should be a figure-of-eight bandage.

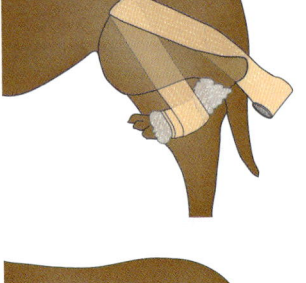

9 Apply a few more layers of conforming gauze bandage to secure the pelvic limb in the flexed position.
10 Apply an adhesive protective bandage material over the conforming bandage to overhang the edge of the conforming gauze to secure the bandage to the skin/fur.

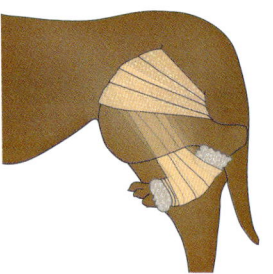

Alternative techniques

■ Ehmer slings are prone to slipping, especially over the cranial aspect of the stifle. These slings can be made using an elastic adhesive bandage alone, with some metatarsal padding. This decreases slipping but the sling is more difficult to remove, and skin irritation is more likely.
■ The sling can also be secured around the abdomen by extending the bandage from the *plantarolateral* aspect of the metatarsus, *lateral* to the flexed pelvic limb and over the *dorsal* aspect of the body, before wrapping it around the abdomen.

Sling maintenance

■ Recommendations for the duration of time for which Ehmer slings need to be maintained to prevent hip reluxation vary: 7 to 10 days is frequently quoted.
■ Ehmer slings must be checked several times daily for complications: ideally every 4 hours.
■ Exercise restriction must be enforced.

Potential complications

- If applied too tightly, potential complications include:
    - Paw swelling due to venous stasis
    - Irritation of the skin, especially over the medial thigh
    - Sloughing of the metatarsal pad
    - Pressure necrosis of the soft tissues
- If the sling becomes wet, moist dermatitis and soft tissue maceration may occur
- Ehmer sling loosening or slipping over the stifle are frequent problems
- Hip re-luxation can also occur due to inappropriate case selection or incorrect technique

Elbow luxation (lateral) – closed reduction

Indications/Use

- Traumatic lateral elbow luxation in the adult dog in the absence of fractures and congenital skeletal deformities
- Closed reduction should be attempted as soon as possible before development of an organized intra-articular haematoma

Contraindications

- Elbow luxation associated with fractures and/or avulsion of ligaments

Equipment

- Radiography equipment

Patient preparation and positioning

- General anaesthesia is required.
- Confirm complete traumatic elbow luxation and rule out associated fractures by palpation and radiography.
- The patient is positioned in lateral recumbency with the affected limb uppermost.

Technique

1 Hold the elbow in complete flexion for a few seconds to fatigue the surrounding muscles.
2 Identify the radial head, semilunar notch of the ulna, and humeral condyles by palpation.
3 Place the elbow in about 110 degrees of flexion. With the carpus flexed to 90 degrees, rotate the antebrachium inward (pronation) using the metacarpal region as a handle. With the thumb of the opposite hand, manipulate the anconeal process toward the lateral epicondyle of the humerus.

4 Apply medial pressure to the olecranon to force the anconeal process medial to the lateral epicondyle. Once this has been achieved, extend the elbow slightly to lock the anconeal process in this position.

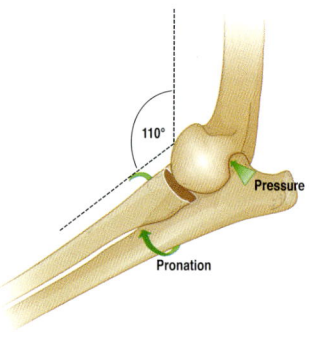

5 Apply medial pressure to the radial head and increase the amount of inward antebrachial rotation. Gradually flex the elbow and adduct the antebrachium simultaneously to force the radial head medially, using the anconeal process as a fulcrum. Slight abduction of the elbow joint may help.

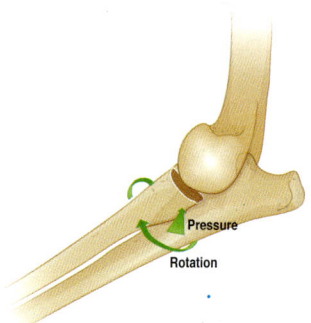

6 Successful reduction is usually accompanied by a dramatic return to a normal range of joint motion and restoration of normal anatomical relationships.

7 Confirm reduction by radiography.

8 Assess the integrity of the collateral ligaments of the elbow using Campbell's test. Flex both the elbow and carpus to 90 degrees and, grasping the paw, check the maximum degree of pronation and supination of the antebrachium.

- Tearing of the medial collateral ligament increases pronation from a normal range of 17–41 to 60–100 degrees.
- Tearing of the lateral collateral ligament increases supination from a normal range of 31–67 to 70–140 degrees.
- If the elbow is unstable with Campbell's test, surgical elbow stabilization should be considered.

9 If the elbow is stable with Campbell's test, apply a **Spica splint** for 2 weeks, followed by 2–4 weeks of rest. A gradual return to normal exercise would then be recommended.

Potential complications

- Re-luxation of the elbow joint
- Decreased range of motion
- Progressive osteoarthritis

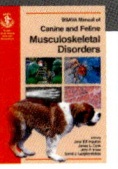

Electrocardiography

Indications/Use

- Detection of an arrhythmia during clinical examination
- As part of the investigation of heart disease
- As part of the investigation of pericardial disease, and for monitoring during pericardiocentesis
- Investigation of collapse, weakness, or exercise intolerance
- Evaluation of cardiac therapy
- Evaluation of trauma cases
- Suspected electrolyte abnormality, particularly hyperkalaemia
- Monitoring during anaesthesia or in a critical-care setting

Equipment

- Electrocardiograph
- Limb leads x4
- Non-traumatic alligator or other clips (with teeth filed down) or disposable pre-gelled self-adhesive electrodes
- Adhesive tape
- ECG gel
- 70% surgical spirit

Patient preparation and positioning

- The animal should be calm and relaxed, before being placed on a surface that is electrically insulated, such as a rubber mat or thick blanket.
- Dogs should ideally be placed in right lateral recumbency, with the fore- and hindlimbs as perpendicular to the long axis of the body as possible. However, in cats, body position appears to be less important.

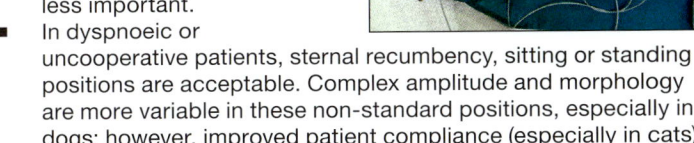

- In dyspnoeic or uncooperative patients, sternal recumbency, sitting or standing positions are acceptable. Complex amplitude and morphology are more variable in these non-standard positions, especially in dogs; however, improved patient compliance (especially in cats)

may produce a better quality trace with fewer artefacts.
- Chemical restraint may cause changes in rhythm, but can be used as a last resort if the alternative is an uninterpretable trace.
- When using non-traumatic alligator or other clips, it is not necessary to remove hair before attaching them.
- Disposable pre-gelled self-adhesive electrodes are applied directly to the pads without previous preparation. However, a wandering baseline and reduced trace quality are more likely to be observed when self-adhesive electrodes are used.

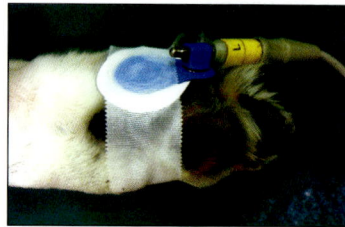

Technique

ECG leads

- The electrodes may be colour-coded and marked for use on human patients. They are attached to the limbs as follows:

Lead	Attachment site	Colour
RA ('right arm')	Right elbow	Red
LA ('left arm')	Left elbow	Yellow
F or LL ('left leg')	Left stifle	Green
N or RL ('right leg', earth lead)	Right stifle	Black

- For routine short ECG, the electrodes are usually attached to the animal using non-traumatic alligator clips. The clips are generally placed on the skin overlying bony protuberances, to minimize the effect of muscle interference. They are then sprayed with surgical spirit or covered in ECG gel to achieve good electrical conductivity.
- Limb electrodes are usually positioned fairly near to the body to reduce movement artefact, using the relatively hairless areas of skin just behind both elbows and in front of the left stifle. Hindlimb electrodes may also be attached to the skin overlying the gastrocnemius tendon.
- The neutral electrode may be placed anywhere, but is usually placed in front of the right stifle.

ECG machine controls

- Sensitivity control: allows the operator to vary the number of centimetres on the paper that are equivalent to 1 mV. Most traces are recorded at 1 cm/mV, but if the complexes are so tall that they cannot be accommodated, decreasing the sensitivity will give a readable trace.

- Paper speed control: allows the operator to choose how quickly the trace is run, usually either 25 or 50 mm/s. Slow running may be useful to save paper in a long recording if looking for intermittent arrhythmias. The trace should be run at a fast paper speed for an animal with a fast heart rate or tachyarrhythmia.
- Filter: allows artefacts to be suppressed, evening out the trace. Its use often causes a marked decrease in the height of the QRS complexes, and this should be taken into account when the trace is interpreted.
- Lead selector: manual lead selection is preferred and the operator should select the six frontal plane leads (Lead I, II, III, aVR, aVL and aVF) in turn.

Recording

1 Once the patient is positioned and the leads attached, switch on the unit and check the sensitivity and paper speed.

2 Ensure that the sensitivity (vertical axis scale) is set to optimize complex size to a height that is clearly seen, without overlapping of leads, and fits the paper.

3 The filter should be turned off.

4 Normally at least five good quality complexes should be recorded in all four leads at 50 mm/s.

5 For rhythm analysis, record a longer (20–30 seconds) lead II strip at 25 mm/s.

6 If intermittent arrhythmias are suspected, it may be necessary to record for several minutes with lead II at 25 mm/s.

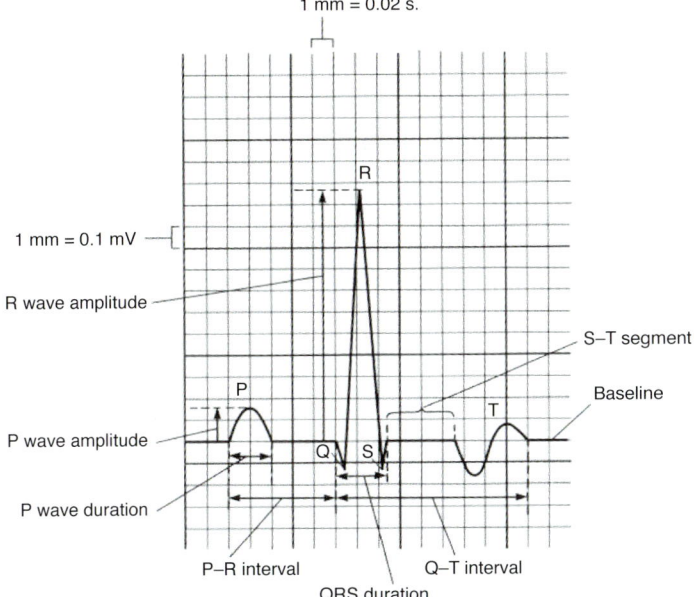

Lead II at 1 cm/mV and 50 mm/s

Reference ranges

Parameter	Unit	Dogs	Cats
Heart rate	beats per minute	70–160 for adult dogs 60–140 for giant breeds up to 180 for toy breeds up to 220 for puppies	120–240
P wave duration	seconds	<0.04 (<0.05 in giant breeds)	<0.04
P wave amplitude	mV	<0.4	<0.2
P–R interval	seconds	0.06–0.13	0.05–0.09
QRS duration	seconds	<0.06	<0.04
R wave amplitude	mV	<2.5–3.0	<0.9
Q–T interval	seconds	0.15–0.25	0.12–0.18
Mean electrical axis (MEA)	degrees	+40 to +100	0 to +160

Data from Tilley LP (1992) *Essentials of Canine and Feline Electrocardiography: Interpretation and Management, 3rd edition.* Philadelphia, Lea & Febiger

Endoscopy of the gastrointestinal tract – (a) upper tract

Indications/Use

- Investigation of clinical signs of oesophageal, gastric and small intestinal (primarily duodenal) disease
- Investigation of radiographic or ultrasonographic abnormalities of the upper gastrointestinal (GI) tract
- Collecting samples from the upper GI tract

Contraindications

- Suspicion of oesophageal or gastric perforation
- Inadequate investigation prior to endoscopy

Equipment

- Flexible endoscope: diameter 7–9 mm; insertion tube at least 1 m long (1.5 m in giant breeds of dog); 4-way tip deflection; minimum 2.2 mm biopsy channel
- Endoscopic viewing equipment
- Facilities for suction and washing the lens
- Flexible endoscopic biopsy forceps
- Mouth gag
- Water-soluble lubricant (e.g. K-Y jelly)
- Container of 10% neutral buffered formalin
- Hypodermic needle: 21 G
- Tissue cassette with foam insert (e.g. CellSafe frames)

Patient preparation and positioning

> **NOTE**
>
> *Do not* perform barium studies at least *24 hours* prior to upper gastrointestinal endoscopy.

- Food must be withheld from *at least 12 (ideally 24) hours prior* to the procedure.
- Water should be withheld from *4 hours prior* to the procedure.
- If delayed gastric emptying is suspected, take a plain lateral radiograph prior to anaesthesia to ensure the stomach and small intestines are empty. If preparation is inadequate, withhold food for a further 12–24 hours.
- **General anaesthesia is essential.** The endotracheal (ET) tube should be tied to the *mandible*, not the maxilla. Avoid atropine if possible, as it affects both motility and secretions of the gastrointestinal tract.
- Place a mouth gag to avoid damage to the endoscope.
- The patient should be positioned in left lateral recumbency, with the head and neck extended.

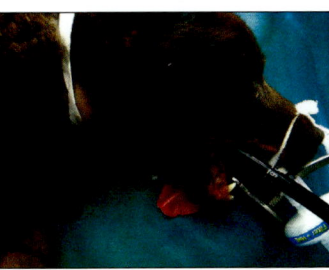

Technique

1 Lubricate the tip of the endoscope with K-Y jelly, avoiding the lens.

2 Pass the endoscope along the midline of the hard palate into the pharynx, reaching the upper oesophageal sphincter.

3 Apply gentle pressure to pass the sphincter.

4 Advance the endoscope in short segments down the **oesophagus** whilst insufflating with air. Try to keep the entire mucosal circumference in view at all times. A better view of the oesophagus will be obtained at the end of the procedure while the endoscope is withdrawn.

5 Pass the endoscope until the gastro-oesophageal junction is visualized, usually seen as a star- or slit-like opening.

6 Align the tip of the endoscope with the lower oesophageal sphincter and gently advance, overcoming slight resistance.

7 If the lower oesophageal sphincter is closed, slightly angle the tip (30 degrees), with continued insufflation, to pass into the stomach.

8 Once inside the **stomach**, inflate with moderate amounts of air to allow orientation. The initial view on entering the stomach is of the junction of the fundus and the body on the greater curvature.

9 If duodenoscopy is to be performed, the stomach should be examined *after* examination of the **duodenum**. Delay in intubating the pylorus can make pyloric intubation more difficult.

10 Follow the rugal folds toward the antrum. Once in the antrum there are few rugal folds, the mucosa is paler in colour and the lumen tapers toward the pylorus. A ring of contraction passing toward the pylorus is also often present.

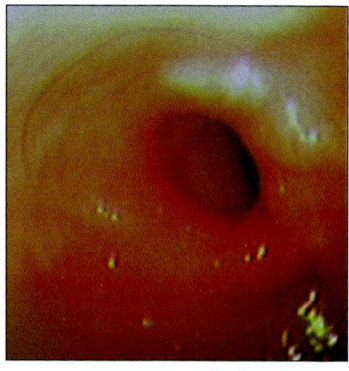

Pyloric sphincter viewed from antrum

PARADOXICAL MOVEMENT

In larger dogs, as the endoscope approaches the antrum, there is a tendency either for the tip to get stuck in the greater curvature or, as the endoscope is advanced, the tip may appear to move backwards, i.e. away from the pylorus.

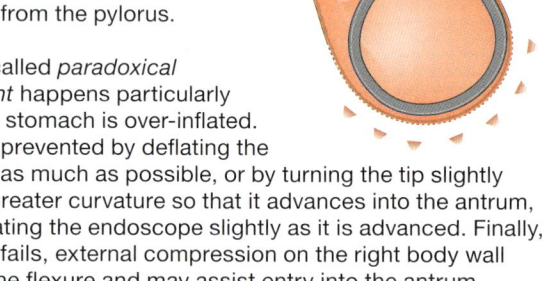

This so-called *paradoxical movement* happens particularly when the stomach is over-inflated. It can be prevented by deflating the stomach as much as possible, or by turning the tip slightly into the greater curvature so that it advances into the antrum, or by rotating the endoscope slightly as it is advanced. Finally, if all else fails, external compression on the right body wall flattens the flexure and may assist entry into the antrum.

11 Position the tip of the endoscope against the pylorus. Maintain this pressure until the next antral contraction and the endoscope may be 'accepted' into the pylorus.

MANOEUVRES TO AID PYLORIC INTUBATION

- Deflate the stomach as much as possible.
- Rotate the endoscope around its long axis.
- Position the patient on its back or in right lateral recumbency. This is best done with the endoscope already positioned in the antrum, as orientation can be more difficult once the animal is repositioned.
- Pass biopsy forceps 'blindly' through the pylorus and then pass the endoscope along this temporary 'guide wire'. However, there is a risk of GI perforation with this technique, and so it should be performed with great care.

12 'Red out' occurs as the endoscope passes into the pyloric canal. The colour will change from 'red out' to 'yellow out', indicating the presence of bile in the duodenum.

13 As the endoscope is passed into the duodenum, angle the tip downwards and to the right.

14 Once in the duodenum, stop advancing the endoscope and inflate with air.

15 Once the duodenum has been examined, return the endoscope to the stomach.

16 Inflate the stomach to allow a complete examination.

17 Retroflex the endoscope (the so-called 'J manoeuvre') to allow visualization of the cardia, which lies in the 'blind spot' on entry to the stomach.

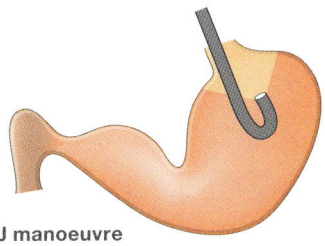

J manoeuvre

18 Deflate the stomach at the end of the procedure and withdraw the endoscope slowly, whilst examining the oesophagus.

Biopsy and sample handling

■ Samples should be collected from:
  ▪ The gastric fundus (take at least 2)
  ▪ The body of the stomach (take at least 4)
  ▪ The antral canal (take at least 2)
  ▪ The periphery of any ulcer
  ▪ Different areas of the duodenum (take 8–10).

> **NOTE**
>
> If pyloric intubation is impossible, the duodenum can still be sampled, *with care*, by passing the forceps 'blindly' through the pylorus. However, it is *unsafe* to take *repeated* samples from the same site without being able to view it.

■ **Samples should always be taken, even if no lesions are apparent.**

1 Position the endoscope in the region to be sampled.

2 Pass the biopsy forceps down the biopsy channel of the endoscope, with the cup firmly closed.

3 Pass the forceps out of the end of the endoscope, open the cup, position on to the mucosa, and close the cup.

4 Withdraw the biopsy forceps through the biopsy channel of the endoscope with the cup firmly closed.

> ### PRACTICAL TIPS
>
> - Position the biopsy forceps perpendicular to the mucosa whenever possible. This will maximize sample collection
> - Avoid overinflation, as this stretches the mucosa and smaller samples will be obtained.
> - Advance the forceps until the mucosa 'tents' and then close them.

5   To remove the samples from the biopsy forceps, immerse in 10% neutral buffered formalin. Then rinse the forceps well in saline before reinserting them into the endoscope.
Alternatively, carefully remove samples from the biopsy forceps with a needle and place directly into formalin or lay on the foam insert of a tissue cassette ('cell-safe' frame).

Potential complications

- Gastrointestinal perforation is rare, but can result from forceful insertion of the endoscope, especially when attempting duodenal intubation. Excessive insufflation can also rupture ulcerated areas
- Significant haemorrhage is rare. Minor and clinically insignificant haemorrhage is very common
- To avoid gastric dilatation, air should be removed from the stomach after gastroscopy
- Overdistension of the stomach causes compression of the caudal vena cava and a drop in venous return. Compression of the diaphragm may also result in decreased tidal volume
- Acute bradycardia most commonly occurs when the duodenum is entered, especially in toy breeds or in patients with severe gastrointestinal disease

Endoscopy of the gastrointestinal tract – (b) lower tract

Indications/Use

- Investigation of clinical signs of lower gastrointestinal tract disease
- Investigation of radiographic or ultrasonographic abnormalities of the lower gastrointestinal (GI) tract
- Collecting samples from the lower GI tract

Contraindications

- Inadequate investigation prior to endoscopy

Equipment

- As for **Endoscopy of the gastrointestinal tract – upper tract** (mouth gag not required)
- *Alternatively,* a rigid endoscope can be used, as this allows excellent visualization of the mucosa, though only of the distal colon and rectum
- Bowel cleansing solution, e.g. Klean-Prep, Moviprep, Dulcobalance
- Equipment for giving an enema, e.g. Higginson's pump

Patient preparation and positioning

- Food must be withdrawn from *at least 24 hours prior* to the procedure.
- Ideally, a bowel cleansing solution (dogs: 22–33 ml/kg by stomach tube, two or three times, at least 4 hours apart; cats: 22–33 ml/kg by **naso-oesophageal tube**) should be administered *12–24 hours prior to* the procedure.
- *Two* warm water enemas should be given on the morning of the procedure, with the last one approximately *1–2 hours* before the procedure. A maximum volume of 15 ml/kg should be administered, using a Higginson's pump or equivalent. **A rectal examination must first be performed, to make sure it is safe to insert the enema tubing.**
- Water should be withheld *from 4 hours prior to* the procedure.
- If inadequate preparation is suspected, take a plain lateral radiograph prior to anaesthesia. If preparation is inadequate, repeat the above steps.
- **General anaesthesia is essential.** Atropine should be avoided if possible, as it affects both motility and secretions of the gastrointestinal tract.
- The patient should be positioned in left lateral recumbency.

Technique

1. Lightly lubricate the distal 20 cm of the endoscope, taking care to avoid the lens.
2. Insert the endoscope gently through the anus and into the **rectum**.
3. Once in the rectum, inflate with air to enable the mucosa to be visualized. Pinching the anus will prevent air escaping.

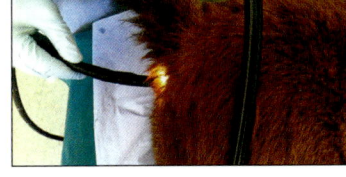

4. Pass the endoscope along the descending **colon**, while insufflating with air.
5. At the cranial end of the descending colon, the junction between the descending and transverse colons (splenic flexure) will be encountered as an obvious 'bend'. The tip of the endoscope should be moved in the direction of the bend and advanced slowly. Some resistance may be felt, but excessive pressure

should not be needed, and could result in rupture of the colon. It is not uncommon to induce 'red-out' whilst doing this.

6   Once in the transverse colon, an image of the mucosa should be re-established.

7   The next 'bend' marks the junction of the transverse and ascending colon; manoeuvre the endoscope in the direction of the bend and advance slowly, as before. Gently moving the endoscope backwards and forwards, while inflating with air, can aid its passage.

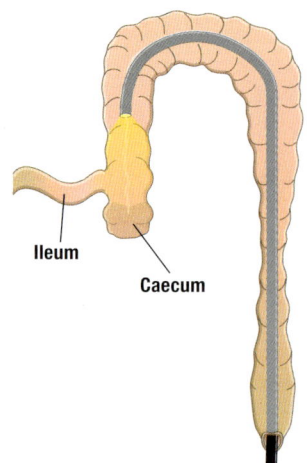

8   The ascending colon is short and ends at the ileocolic junction. This is recognized by the adjacent blind-ending sac, the caecum.

9   Carefully examine the **caecum**.

10 Withdraw the endoscope slowly and take biopsy samples. It is often easier to examine and sample the colon while the endoscope is being withdrawn.

Biopsy and sample handling

■ Samples should be collected from:
  ■ Ascending and transverse colon (take 2 or 3 from each)
  ■ Descending colon (take 4 or 5).
■ **Samples should always be taken, even if no lesions are apparent.**

1   Position the endoscope in the region to be sampled.

2   Pass the biopsy forceps down the biopsy channel of the endoscope, with the cup firmly closed.

3   Pass the forceps out of the end of the endoscope, open the cup, position on to the mucosa, and close the cup.

4   Withdraw the biopsy forceps through the biopsy channel of the endoscope with the cup firmly closed.

PRACTICAL TIPS

■ Position the biopsy forceps perpendicular to the mucosa whenever possible. This will maximize sample collection

■ Avoid overinflation, as this stretches the mucosa and smaller samples will be obtained.

■ Advance the forceps until the mucosa 'tents' and then close them.

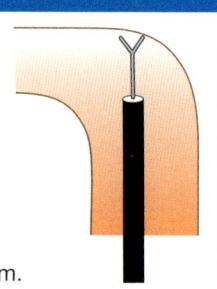

5 To remove the samples from the biopsy forceps, immerse in 10% neutral buffered formalin. Then rinse the forceps well in saline before reinserting them into the endoscope.
Alternatively, carefully remove samples from the biopsy forceps with a needle and place directly into formalin or lay on the foam insert of a tissue cassette ('cell-safe' frame).

Potential complications

- Gastrointestinal perforation is rare, but can result from forceful insertion of the endoscope. Excessive insufflation can also rupture ulcerated areas. Exploratory surgery is required if either of these occur
- Significant haemorrhage is rare. Minor and clinically insignificant haemorrhage is very common

> **FURTHER INFORMATION**
>
> Further information on endoscopy of the GI tract can be found in the *BSAVA Manual of Canine and Feline Endoscopy and Endosurgery.*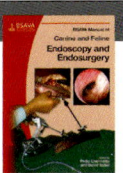

Endotracheal wash

Indications/Use

- To obtain a sample from the airways for cytology and bacteriology
- Generally yields samples representative of the trachea and primary or (at best) secondary bronchi, although some material from the lower bronchioles and alveoli may be collected

> **OPTIONS**
>
> - The upper airway of medium-sized and large dogs may also be sampled by **transtracheal wash**.
> - The lower airways of dogs and cats may be sampled using **bronchoalveolar lavage**.

Contraindications

- Compromised respiratory function
- Patients with pulmonary parenchymal disease, rather than tracheal or bronchial disease

Equipment

- Sterile endotracheal (ET) tube
- Male dog urinary catheter (4–6 Fr). The tip of the catheter can be

cut off to remove the side holes, but care must be taken to ensure that the tip is not sharp
- Topical local anaesthetic spray
- Warmed 0.9% sterile saline
- 10 ml and 20 ml syringes
- 3-way tap
- Sterile plain and EDTA collection tubes
- Microscope slides

Patient preparation and positioning

- Preoxygenate the patient using a face mask prior to induction of general anaesthesia.
- General anaesthesia is essential.
- The patient is placed in either lateral or sternal recumbency.

SPECIAL CONSIDERATIONS FOR CATS

Extra care should be taken when performing an endotracheal wash in cats, as their airways are particularly prone to bronchospasm.

- The procedure should be performed as quickly as possible, with the minimum of trauma.
- To reduce the risk of bronchospasm, terbutaline can be given approximately 30 minutes pre-bronchoscopy (0.015 mg/kg s.c. or i.m). Onset of action is 15–30 minutes and is usually notable by an increase in heart rate.
- Terbutaline should also be available for giving during the procedure if bronchospasm still occurs.

Technique

1 The urinary catheter will be passed into the trachea through the ET tube. Pre-measure the length of the catheter needed to reach the tracheal bifurcation (approximately the 4th intercostal space), and mark this on the packaging.

2 If intubating a cat, apply topical local anaesthetic spray to the larynx.

3 Insert a sterile ET tube into the trachea, avoiding oral contamination.

NOTE

Take care to minimize contact between the tip of the ET tube and the oropharynx during intubation, to avoid oropharyngeal contamination.

---

4 Pass the sterile catheter down the ET tube to the pre-marked length. To avoid contamination, the catheter should be inserted by feeding it *through the sterile packaging.*

5 Attach a 3-way tap to the catheter.

6   Inject warmed sterile saline (0.5 ml/kg) into the catheter via the 3-way tap.

7   Immediately aspirate back the saline.

8   Repeat the injection of saline and the aspiration two or three times as required. A total recovery of 1–3 ml of a slightly turbid fluid with a foamy layer at the top (representative of surfactant) represents good sample recovery. Coupage and turning the patient may improve cell yield.

9   Following completion of an endotracheal wash, continue administration of 100% oxygen and volatile agent for 5 minutes, to allow time to detect any immediate complications of the procedure, e.g. bronchospasm. Continue oxygen supplementation via the ET tube until extubation. Pulse oximetry should be utilized to measure the patient's oxygenation throughout the recovery from anaesthesia, and during the postoperative procedure.

Sample handling

- Submit a portion of the sample in a sterile plain tube for culture.
- Place an aliquot in an EDTA tube for cytology.
- The cells collected are fragile, so samples should be processed as soon as possible. If samples are to be sent to an external laboratory, fresh air-dried unstained smears of any flocculent/mucoid material should also be made (see **Fine needle aspiration**). Direct smears of the fluid can also be made, but most samples are poorly cellular.

Potential complications

- Bronchospasm
- Laryngospasm and coughing
- Haemorrhage
- Iatrogenic infection

FURTHER INFORMATION

Details on cytology of upper respiratory tract samples can be found in the *BSAVA Manual of Canine and Feline Clinical Pathology*.

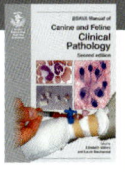

Fine needle aspiration

Indications/Use

- To obtain a sample for cytology. Some tissues or lesions give much better cell yields and/or greater chance of a definitive diagnosis

Contraindications

- Coagulopathy

> **WARNING**
> - **Clotting times (APTT and OSPT) should ideally be checked before aspirating masses associated with the liver, spleen, kidney or other well vascularized organs.**

Equipment

- As required for **Aseptic preparation – (a) non-surgical procedures**
- Hypodermic needles: 23 G; ¾ to 3 inch (depending on depth of tissue to be sampled)
- 5 ml syringe
- Microscope slides
- Hairdryer
- Ultrasound equipment (where required)

Patient preparation and positioning

- Fine needle aspiration of superficial masses can usually be performed with the patient under physical restraint or light sedation.
- Fine needle aspiration of abdominal viscera or masses may require heavy sedation or general anaesthesia.
- The animal is positioned with the area to be sampled uppermost.
- **Aseptic preparation – (a) non-surgical procedures** is performed on the skin over the site to be aspirated, or the skin overlying the needle insertion site (for abdominal viscera/mass aspiration).

Technique

1 For superficial masses, immobilize the mass with one hand and insert the needle into the lesion using the other hand. For deep masses, or those within the abdomen or thorax, immobilization is usually not possible.

2 Aspiration may be performed using the 'needle-only' method or by using continuous suction.

- **Needle-only method:** This method is useful for aspirating soft masses/lesions and lymph nodes. It has the advantages that fragile cells are not damaged by suction, and haemodilution is minimized.

i   Insert the needle into the lesion without a syringe attached.
ii Gently redirect the needle within the lesion to gather a core of cells in the barrel of the needle.
iii Remove the needle from the lesion.

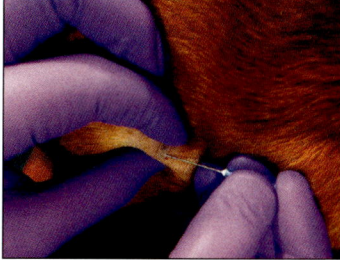

- **Continuous suction method:** This method is useful for aspirating firm masses such as soft tissue sarcomas, which tend not to exfoliate cells well. It can, however, cause more damage to fragile cells and may increase blood contamination.

i   Insert the needle into the lesion with a 5 ml syringe attached.
ii With the needle in the lesion, withdraw the plunger to one-half to three-quarters of the volume of the syringe (to apply 2–3 ml suction).

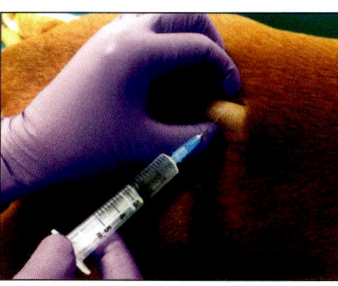

iii Maintain suction and move the needle to and fro, redirecting the needle several times within the lesion.
iv Release the suction and remove the needle from the mass.
v   Disconnect the needle from the syringe.

3 Attach an air-filled syringe to the needle.
4 Expel the contents of the needle containing the sample on to one or more clean microscope slides and prepare smears using one of the techniques described below.

Ultrasound guidance

Fine needle aspiration from internal organs and from intra-thoracic or intra-abdominal masses is best performed under ultrasound guidance.

- Care should be taken to remove excess ultrasound gel from the area of skin through which the needle is to be inserted, as gel can obscure cellular detail and alter the staining characteristics of the sample.
- The needle should be introduced close to the ultrasound probe, to make visualization and tracking of the needle point easier.
- Although a one-handed active aspiration technique with a syringe attached is possible, in many cases introducing the needle alone and redirecting its path within the area of interest is not only adequate but easier if single-handed.

Sample handling

Squash preparation

With experience, this technique produces excellent smears. However, in inexperienced hands cells may be damaged/ruptured, resulting in an unreadable smear.

1 Expel the aspirate on to the centre of a microscope slide.
2 Place a second spreader slide horizontally and at right angles to spread the sample, taking care not to exert downward pressure that could rupture the cells.
3 Using only the surface tension between the two slides, draw the spreader slide quickly and smoothly across the bottom slide.
4 Rapidly dry the smear by waving it in the air or under a hairdryer. **Note that it is the smear produced on the *underside of the spreader slide* that will be examined.**

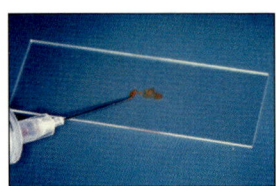

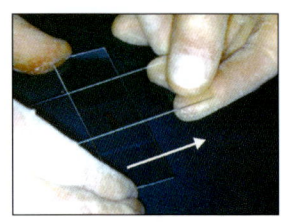

Blood film technique

This technique has less potential for causing cell rupture, and is useful for lymph node aspirates since lymphocytes are fragile. It is *not* suitable for samples of low cellularity, e.g. fluid aspirates. A 'spreader' slide with one corner missing is used to prepare the smear in order to avoid spreading the cells over the edges of the slide.

1 Expel the aspirate near to one end of a microscope slide in the centre line.
2 Hold the 'spreader' between the thumb and middle finger, placing the index finger on top of the 'spreader'.
3 Place the 'spreader' in front of the aspirate, at an angle of about 30 degrees, and draw it backwards until it comes into contact with the sample, allowing the sample to spread out rapidly along the edge of the 'spreader'.
4 Advance the 'spreader' forwards smoothly and quickly.
5 After the 'spreader' has been advanced two-thirds of the way along the bottom slide, lift it abruptly upwards in order to concentrate cells at the end of the smear.
6 Rapidly dry the smear by waving it in the air or under a hairdryer.

Potential complications

- Haemorrhage. Any haemorrhage should be controlled by firm pressure over the site for several minutes. Continued haemorrhage from an internal organ is an indication for exploratory surgery
- Tissue damage

Gall bladder aspiration

Indications/Use

- Investigation of biliary tract disease
- To obtain samples for cytology and bacteriology

Contraindications

- Biliary tract obstruction, as this may result in leakage or rupture
- Severe disease of the gall bladder wall, as this may result in leakage or rupture

Equipment

- As required for **Aseptic preparation – (a) non-surgical procedures**
- Ultrasound machine (for ultrasound-guided aspiration)
- 10–20 ml syringe
- Hypodermic or spinal needles: 21–23 G; 1.5 to 3 inches (depending on depth of the gall bladder)
- EDTA and sterile plain collection tubes

Patient preparation and positioning

APPROACH

Gall bladder aspiration is performed under ultrasound guidance or at the time of an exploratory laparotomy. When performed under ultrasound guidance, a transhepatic approach is used to minimize leakage of bile. Gall bladder aspiration should never be performed 'blind'.

CLOTTING TESTS

If to be performed under ultrasound guidance, a coagulation panel (prothrombin and activated partial thromboplastin times) should be performed prior to gall bladder aspiration. If coagulation abnormalities are found, vitamin K (1.0 mg/kg s.c. q12h) should be given for 24 hours before aspiration, and repeat coagulation testing performed to confirm correction prior to aspiration. If vitamin K has no effect, a **blood transfusion** (or ideally a transfusion of fresh plasma) should be performed, with coagulation testing then repeated before aspiration is carried out. Provided no coagulation abnormalities are detected, aspiration should be performed as soon as possible after a blood transfusion.

- If performed under ultrasound guidance, general anaesthesia or heavy sedation is essential.
- The patient is placed in dorsal or lateral recumbency, depending on which position allows optimal visualization of the liver and gall bladder.
- Using ultrasonography, the optimal site for gall bladder aspiration is identified. This is often on the left side of the patient as this is more likely to allow the needle to be inserted through adjacent liver tissue prior to entry into the gall bladder. In large dogs, an intercostal approach may be required.
- **Aseptic preparation – (a) non-surgical procedures** is performed on the skin over a wide area around the site of needle entry.

Technique

1. If using ultrasonography, the site previously identified is used. If performed during surgery, identify a site in the body of the gall bladder and away from its neck; there is no need to use a transhepatic approach, as the site of needle insertion can be monitored for leakage.
2. Insert the needle with the syringe attached into the gall bladder, ideally at an angle of approximately 45 degrees to the body wall. This will help to minimize leakage of bile following withdrawal of the needle.
3. Aspirate bile into the syringe, removing as much as possible in order to minimize leakage after needle removal.
4. Monitor for bile leakage for approximately 5–10 minutes after aspiration, either visually at the time of surgery or with ultrasonography.
5. If evidence of significant bile leakage, an exploratory laparotomy is required.

> **WARNING**
>
> - It should be remembered that there is still a risk of haemorrhage even if coagulation parameters are normal, and it is important to have the option of prompt surgical intervention in case of complications. The animal also needs to be kept under close observation after the procedure and monitored for evidence of haemorrhage (e.g. tachycardia, pallor, weakness, reduced pulse quality).

Sample handling

- Submit a portion of the sample in a sterile plain tube for culture.
- Place an aliquot in an EDTA tube for cytology.

Potential complications

- Leakage of bile, leading to bile peritonitis
- Gall bladder rupture
- Haemorrhage

Gastric decompression – (a) orogastric intubation

Indications/Use

- Stabilization of dogs with gastric dilatation and volvulus (GDV) prior to surgery
- Orogastric intubation is superior to percutaneous needle decompression (see below)

> **WARNING**
> - **Fluid therapy for the treatment of hypovolaemic shock must be initiated prior to gastric decompression.**

Equipment

- Wide-bore stomach tube
- 7.5 cm wide roll of adhesive bandage with a hollow plastic core
- Funnel
- Bucket
- Warmed normal (0.9%) saline, lactated Ringer's (Hartmann's) solution or tap water

Patient preparation and positioning

- Sedation may be required to reduce anxiety, but monitor for hypotension.
- A right lateral abdominal radiograph should be obtained to confirm the diagnosis of GDV if there is any doubt.
- The patient should be on a table or trolley to allow gravity to aid in gastric emptying.
- A 'sitting' position or sternal recumbency is often best, but gastric decompression may be achieved in right lateral recumbency.

Technique

1 Mark the distance from the dog's nose to its 11th rib on the stomach tube. The tube should not be passed beyond this length, to minimize the risk of rupture of a potentially compromised gastric wall.
2 Insert the bandage roll longitudinally into the dog's mouth. The mouth is held closed around the bandage roll by an assistant or by applying tape around the dog's muzzle.
3 Insert the stomach tube through the core of the bandage roll and gently down into the dog's stomach. Rotating the stomach tube gently about its long axis may aid passage through the gastro-oesophageal junction.
4 Gaseous decompression is achieved spontaneously.

5 Further emptying of the stomach can be achieved by lavage with copious volumes of warm saline, lactated Ringer's or tap water.

i Pour the solution from a height into the stomach, using a funnel attached to the end of the stomach tube.

ii Allow stomach contents to flow out of the stomach by lowering the tube below the level of the dog.

Potential complications

- Trauma to the gastro-oesophageal junction
- Passage of the stomach tube through a compromised gastric wall

Gastric decompression – (b) percutaneous needle

Indications/Use

- May facilitate orogastric intubation
- Should be performed when orogastric intubation is not possible

Equipment

- As for **Aseptic preparation – (a) non-surgical procedures**
- 16 or 18 G over-the-needle intravenous catheter

Patient preparation and positioning

- Sedation may be required to reduce anxiety, but monitor for hypotension.
- A right lateral abdominal radiograph should be obtained to confirm the diagnosis of GDV if there is any doubt.
- The patient is placed in left lateral or sternal recumbency.
- **Aseptic preparation – (a) non-surgical procedures** of an area of skin over the most distended part of the right abdominal wall.

Technique

1 Percuss the right abdominal wall and define the site of greatest tympany, where the distended stomach is likely to be directly abutting the abdominal wall.

2 Insert the catheter percutaneously directly into the stomach.

3 Remove the stylet of the catheter to allow air to escape freely from the stomach.

Potential complications

- Entry of the catheter into another abdominal organ

Gastric decontamination

Indications/Use
- In most cases of acute toxin ingestion

> **METHOD SELECTION**
> - Gastric decontamination is performed either by induction of **emesis** or by **gastric lavage**. Gastric lavage is not as effective as emesis, so if emesis can be safely induced this is preferred.
> - Activated charcoal should be administered following emesis/gastric lavage; it acts as an adsorbent for many toxins and further reduces GI absorption. However, activated charcoal may be contraindicated if orally administered/treatments or antidotes are to be given.

Contraindications
- Substance was ingested more than 2–3 hours prior to presentation (seek advice after this time as some substances may still be retrieved after this period)
- **Emesis induction** should not be performed:
    - If the ingested substance was caustic or corrosive, due to the risk of further damage to the oesophagus
    - If ingesta contain paraffin, petroleum products or other oily or volatile organic compounds, due to risk of inhalation
    - If the patient is unconscious, fitting, in respiratory distress, or unable to stand

Equipment
- An **emetic** agent such as apomorphine, an alpha-2 agonist (e.g. xylazine or medetomidine) or sodium carbonate (washing soda)
- For **gastric lavage**: equipment as for Gastric decompression – (a) orogastric intubation (adhesive bandage not required)
- Activated charcoal

Patient preparation and positioning
- For the induction of **emesis**, patients should be conscious and standing.
- For **gastric lavage**, the patient should be lightly anaesthetised and the trachea intubated with a cuffed endotracheal tube. The patient should be in lateral or sternal recumbency, ideally with the head at a level below that of the body.

Technique

Induction of emesis
There are different options for the induction of emesis in different species.

Dogs

- Apomorphine 0.02–0.04 mg/kg i.v. (most effective route), s.c. or i.m. (least effective).
- Sodium carbonate (washing soda) crystals. The dose is empirical but usually a large crystal in a medium- to large-breed dog and a small crystal in a small dog. **DO NOT confuse with caustic soda (sodium hydroxide).**

Cats

- Alpha-2 agonists such as xylazine (1–3 mg/kg i.m.) or medetomidine (0.01–0.02 mg/kg i.v., s.c. or i.m.). *Note that these drugs may also result in the unwanted effect of sedation.*
- Sodium carbonate (washing soda) crystals. The dose is empirical but usually a small crystal is appropriate for a cat. **DO NOT confuse with caustic soda (sodium hydroxide).**

> **WARNING**
>
> - **Other options such as syrup of ipecacuanha, household remedies (table salt, mustard) and hydrogen peroxide are not recommended and can be dangerous.**

Gastric lavage

1 Mark the distance from the animal's nose to its 11th rib on the stomach tube. The tube should not be passed beyond this length, to minimize the risk of rupture of a potentially compromised gastric wall.
2 Insert the stomach tube into the animal's mouth, down the oesophagus and into the stomach. Rotating the stomach tube gently about its long axis may aid passage through the gastro-oesophageal junction.
3 Instil approximately 10 ml/kg warmed water, 0.9% saline or lactated Ringer's (Hartmann's).
4 Agitate the animal's stomach by manual palpation.
5 Allow the fluid to drain out of the stomach tube, by lowering the tube and the animal's head.
6 The procedure should be repeated until the fluid returned is relatively clear (commonly 10–20 times).

Administration of activated charcoal

- Activated charcoal is usually given via a stomach tube after gastric lavage, but can also be administered orally after the induction of emesis.
- Slurries of activated charcoal are more effective than tablets or capsules.
- Recommended dose is 0.5–4 g/kg orally and can be repeated every 4–6 hours for the first 24–48 hours, or until charcoal is seen in the faeces.
- Repeat dose administration of activated charcoal is particularly important when the agent is enterohepatically recirculated, e.g. salicylates, barbiturates, theobromine, methylxanthines.

- Activated charcoal can slow gastrointestinal transit time, thus co-administration of a cathartic (e.g. sorbitol or magnesium sulphate) can be considered, although this is not recommended in dehydrated patients or patients where there is a suspicion of ileus.

> **WARNING**
> - **Activated charcoal reduces the absorption of, and therefore the efficacy of, orally administered drugs.**

Potential complications

- Damage to the oesophagus from caustic or corrosive ingesta or the stomach tube
- Inhalation of stomach contents
- Passage of the stomach tube through a damaged gastric wall

Gastrostomy tube placement – (a) endoscopic

Indications/Use

- Long-term (months to years) nutritional support
- Where naso-oesophageal or oesophagostomy tube feeding is not possible (e.g. vomiting, severe oesophageal disease, head/neck trauma)

Contraindications

- Gastric outflow obstruction
- Comatose, recumbent or dysphoric animals that are at risk of aspiration
- Likely temporary anorexia, especially when an alternative feeding method could be used (e.g. **naso-oesophageal tube**, **oesophagostomy tube**)

Equipment

- A commercial PEG (percutaneous endoscopic gastrostomy) kit containing a radiopaque polyurethane 36 inch gastrostomy tube, introducer needle, guidewire, fixation device and Y-adaptor:

  - 16 Fr (cats and small dogs)
  - 20–22 Fr (medium and large dogs)
- Endoscope: 7–10 mm diameter; 1 m long
- Endoscopic grasping or biopsy forceps
- As required for **Aseptic preparation – (a) non-surgical procedures**

- No. 15 or 20 scalpel
- Sterile dressing to cover the tube site
- Tube gauze or loose body wrap

Patient preparation and positioning

- General anaesthesia is required.
- The patient is positioned in right lateral recumbency.
- **Aseptic preparation – (a) non-surgical procedures** is performed on an area on the left flank (approximately 15 cm x 15 cm in a medium-sized dog), extending caudally from the costal arch and dorsoventrally from the transverse processes of the lumbar vertebrae to the level of the ventral end of the 13th rib.

Technique

1 Insert the endoscope down the oesophagus and into the stomach. Insufflate the stomach so it is moderately distended.

2 An assistant applies pressure on the stomach with a finger just behind the last rib, and the endoscopist visualizes the indented mucosa caused. This allows identification of the site into which the tube will be inserted. *Alternatively,* the light of the endoscope may be seen shining through the body wall and used to locate the site of catheter insertion. Ideally, the tube should enter the stomach at the junction of the body and the antrum; if it is too near the pylorus it may cause an obstruction.

3 A 3–5 mm skin incision is made over the site identified for tube insertion.

4 Withdraw the endoscope back into the cardia.

5 Insert the introducer needle percutaneously into the inflated stomach via the skin incision.

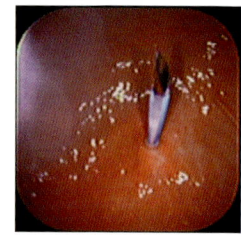

6 Pass endoscopic grasping or biopsy forceps down the biopsy channel and out the end of the endoscope. Open the forceps and position them by the tip of the introducer needle ready to grab the guidewire.

7 Pass the guidewire through the introducer catheter and thread it into the stomach.

8 Grasp the guidewire with the endoscopic grasping or biopsy forceps. Without withdrawing the forceps into the biopsy channel, hold the forceps and endoscope as one unit and slowly pull this out of the stomach, up the oesophagus and out of the mouth. **Keep the forceps closed at all times.**

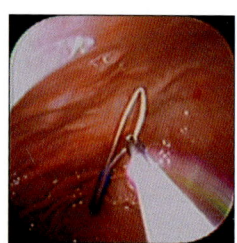

9 Once the tip of the endoscope, forceps and guidewire come out of the animal's mouth, release the guidewire from the forceps.

10 Attach the guidewire to the end of the gastrostomy tube.

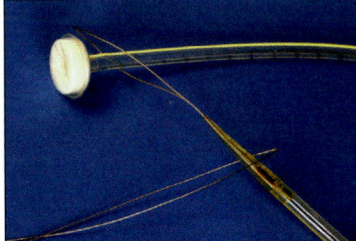

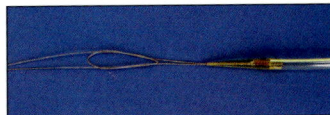

The wire loops are interlocked.

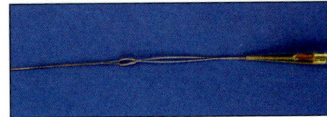

The mushroom tip of the PEG tube is looped through the swaged-on wire loop to join it to the wire loop passing out of the mouth.

Pulling the wires tight produces a knotless connection.

11 Pull the other end of the guidewire, from where it exits the animal's flank, to draw the feeding tube into the mouth, down the oesophagus, into the stomach, and out through the stomach wall. Firm traction is needed to pull the feeding tube through the stomach and body wall layers and out through the skin incision.

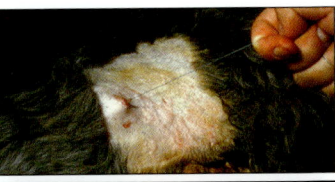

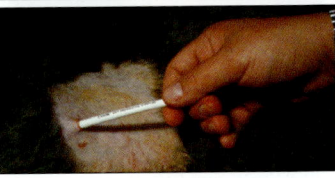

12 Once the gastrostomy tube has exited the body wall, pull it so that the bumper on the end of the tube that is to remain in the stomach lies snugly against the stomach wall.

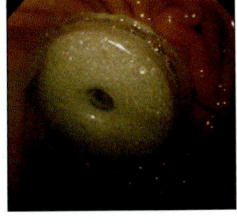

13 Pass the endoscope back into the stomach to check that the tube is positioned in the correct area and that the bumper is flat against the stomach wall.

14 Secure the tube with the fixation device contained within the kit. Note that the tube should not be pulled and fixed excessively tightly, as this could result in skin and stomach wall necrosis.

15 In case of future migration, note the correct position of the tube relative to the body wall, based on the centimetre graduations on the side of the tube.

16 Cut the tube to the desired length. Attach the adaptor contained within the kit on to the end of the tube.

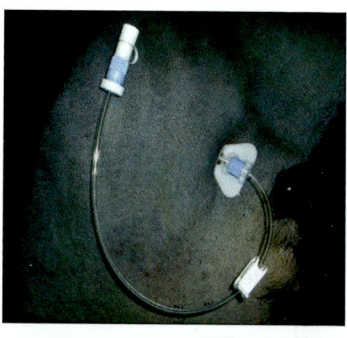

17 Apply a sterile dressing to the skin stoma site.

18 Place tube gauze or a loose body wrap to protect the remaining tube and prevent it from being removed.

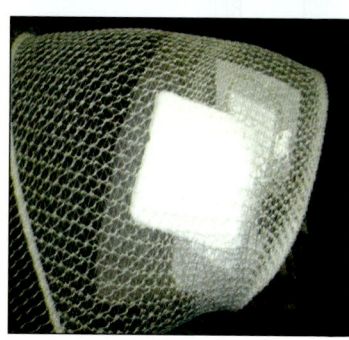

Feeding technique

> **NOTE**
>
> Do not use the tube for the first 24 hours, to allow a primary seal to form between the stomach and body wall.

1 Instil sterile saline initially, in case the tube has migrated. If there is any doubt as to its position, take abdominal radiographs with or without sterile **iodinated contrast medium**.

2 Before feeding each time, flush the tube with small amounts (5–10 ml) of lukewarm tap water.

3 Aspirate the contents of the stomach with an empty syringe prior to feeding. If gastric emptying is delayed and there is more than half the previous meal in the stomach, skip the feed and consider motility modifiers such as metoclopramide.

4 Food should be warmed to body temperature and injected into the tube over approximately 5 minutes.
  - Feed only one third of the resting energy requirement (RER) on the first day.
  - On the second day, feed two-thirds of the RER, increasing to the entire RER on day three.
  - Divide the daily requirement into multiple (5 or 6) feeds per 24 hours.

5 Flush the tube *after every feed* with 5–10 ml of lukewarm tap water.

RER

The resting energy requirement is now used as the 'baseline' energy recommendation for hospitalized dogs and cats, regardless of the disease or surgery.

The following equation can be used to calculate the RER in kcal/day for cats or dogs:

RER = 70 x bodyweight (kg) $^{0.75}$

Alternatively, for animals >2 kg the following equation can be used:

RER = 30 x bodyweight (kg) + 70

Note: To convert kcal to kilojoules (kJ) multiply by 4.185

Tube maintenance and removal

- Inspect and clean the stoma site daily, applying antibiotic cream if necessary.
- If the tube becomes blocked, 3 ml of a carbonated drink (e.g. cola or soda water) can be instilled and left for 5–10 minutes to help dislodge blockages.
- The gastrostomy tube should remain in place for at least 7–10 days before removal. This period of time allows a permanent adhesion to form between the stomach and the body wall, and to prevent leakage of gastric contents into the peritoneal cavity.
- If a gastrostomy tube is accidentally removed before intended, it can be re-placed through the same stoma site if the procedure is performed rapidly (e.g. within 24 hours of the tube removal).
- Commercial PEG tubes have a collapsible soft bumper. To remove the tube, remove the gauze dressing at the skin stoma site and the loose body wrap, and undo the fixation device. Using firm pressure, pull the tube out of the stomach through the skin.

Potential complications

Major complications of feeding tube placement in dogs and cats are uncommon and can usually be avoided with proper technique and careful client counselling.

The most common complications are:

- Tube blockage
- If the tube is not capped, leakage of gastric acid can cause acid burns on the skin
- Infection at the tube site
- Tube dislodgement or removal
- Vomiting following feeding

Other complications include:

- Leakage around the tube site
- Diarrhoea due to overfeeding
- Delayed gastric emptying due to effects of the tube on gastric motility
- Splenic laceration
- Necrosis of the gastric wall if the tube is too tight

FURTHER INFORMATION

Further information on endoscopic placement of gastrostomy tubes can be found in the *BSAVA Manual of Canine and Feline Endoscopy and Endosurgery.*

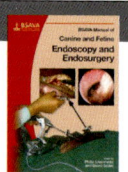

Gastrostomy tube placement – (b) surgical

Indications/Use

- Where a gastrostomy tube is required in a patient undergoing another surgical procedure

Equipment

- Mushroom-tipped catheter with large ('XL') mushroom
  - Cats and small dogs: 16 Fr
  - Dogs: 20–24 Fr
- Gastrostomy tube connector and bung
- As required for **Aseptic preparation – (b) surgical procedures**
- Suture materials
- Soft tissue surgical instrument set

Patient positioning and preparation

- General anaesthesia is required.
- The animal should be placed in right lateral recumbency or in dorsal recumbency.
- **Aseptic preparation – (b) surgical procedures** is required.

Technique

1. The stomach is approached via a left paracostal coeliotomy or a ventral midline coeliotomy.
2. Make a full thickness stab incision in the left abdominal wall just caudal to the costal arch at the level of the fundus of the stomach.

3 Pass the feeding tube half-way through the incision so that the mushroom tip is within the abdomen and the catheter tip outside.

4 Place a full-thickness purse-string suture in the fundus, midway between the lesser and greater curvatures. The diameter of the purse string should be large enough to facilitate passage of the feeding tube through the centre. Do *not* tie the ends of the suture, but hold them with haemostats.

5 Make a stab incision in the centre of the purse-string suture, just large enough to push the folded mushroom tip of the catheter through.

6 Tighten the purse-string suture and secure it around the shaft of the gastrostomy tube; this seals the stomach wall around the tube.

7 Place four horizontal mattress sutures around the feeding tube between the stomach wall and the transversus abdominis muscle in a square configuration, to appose the stomach to the left abdominal wall. Place all the sutures before any is tied.

8 Omentum can be wrapped around the gastropexy site to promote healing.

9 Pull the external (catheter tip) end of the tube so that the mushroom tip is positioned snugly against the stomach wall.

10 Secure the tube to the skin using a Chinese finger-trap suture.

11 Close the coeliotomy wound routinely.

Tube care and maintenance; Feeding technique; Tube removal; Potential complications

As for **Gastrostomy tube placement – (a) endoscopic**.

FURTHER INFORMATION

Further details on placement and use of gastrostomy tubes can be found in the *BSAVA Manual of Canine and Feline Gastroenterology* and the *BSAVA Manual of Canine and Feline Rehabilitation, Supportive and Palliative Care.*

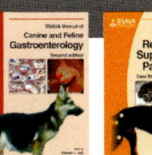

Haemagglutination test

Indications/Use

- Confirmation of suspected immune-mediated haemolytic anaemia (IMHA)

> **NOTES**
>
> - A negative test result does *not* rule out IMHA. The direct antiglobulin or Coombs' test, which detects antibodies associated with the surface or red blood cells, should be performed if IMHA is suspected and autoagglutination cannot be demonstrated.
> - A positive haemagglutination test is regarded as being diagnostic for IMHA and precludes the need to perform the Coombs' test.

Equipment

- 1 ml of venous blood, freshly collected in an EDTA tube (*see* **Blood sampling – (a) venous**)
- Microhaematocrit tube
- Microscope slide and coverslip
- 0.9% saline
- 2 ml syringe and needle
- Microscope

Technique

1 Using a microhaematocrit tube, place 2–4 drops of blood on a microscope slide.
2 Using a syringe and needle, withdraw saline from a bag and add an equal volume to the blood on the slide.
3 Rock the slide gently for 30 seconds.
4 Examine the slide grossly for agglutination, i.e. clumping of red cells.

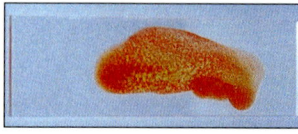

5 Add a coverslip and examine microscopically under high power.
6 A positive result is confirmed by the *microscopic* visualization of clumps of randomly oriented red blood cells.

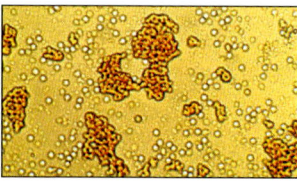

ROULEAUX

It is very important to examine the slide using a microscope, as rouleaux formation appears identical to true agglutination on gross examination. If rouleaux formation persists, add additional saline in an attempt to disperse this natural phenomenon.

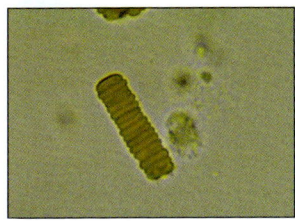 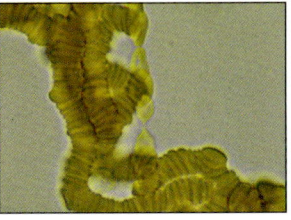

Rouleaux formations

FURTHER INFORMATION

Further details of the test and its interpretation can be found in the *BSAVA Manual of Canine and Feline Clinical Pathology*.

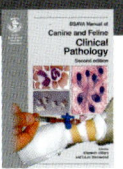

Hip luxation – closed reduction

Indications/Use

■ Recent traumatic hip luxation

Contraindications

■ If luxation has been present for longer than 7–10 days, closed reduction is unlikely to be successful

Equipment

■ Soft cotton rope or towel sling
■ Sandbag
■ As for **Ehmer sling**

Patient preparation and positioning

■ General anaesthesia is required.
■ Ventrodorsal and lateral radiographs of the pelvis should be obtained to confirm hip luxation and to evaluate the direction of the luxation. Radiography is also required to detect avulsion fractures of the teres ligament, chip fractures of the dorsal acetabular rim, other pelvic fractures and the presence of pre-existing coxofemoral osteoarthritis, which may complicate management of hip luxation.

- The patient should be positioned in lateral recumbency, with the affected limb uppermost.
- For large dogs it may be beneficial to secure their hindquarters to the table, using a soft cotton rope placed within the inguinal region of the affected limb and secured caudodorsally to the table. *Alternatively,* the affected pelvic limb may be supported using a towel sling: the towel is passed through the inguinal region and both ends are held by an assistant standing on the dorsal side of the patient.

Technique

Craniodorsal luxation (the majority of cases)

1 Manipulate the femoral head to loosen any adhesions, and apply caudoventral traction to the stifle region to counteract muscle contraction.
2 Extend the leg, adduct and externally rotate it with continued traction to lift the femoral head over the dorsal rim of the acetabulum and reduce the hip. The greater trochanter may be guided caudally and distally with the non-dominant hand.
3 A palpable/audible click may be noted at reduction. Apply pressure to the trochanter and rotate the joint to express any haematoma from the joint space.
4 Manipulate the hip and check it for range of motion and stability.
5 Confirm reduction radiographically.
6 If appropriate, apply an **Ehmer sling** for 7–10 days.

Cranioventral luxation

1 Manipulate the femoral head to the craniodorsal position and reduce as described above.
   Alternatively, it may be possible to manipulate the femoral head directly back into the acetabulum by palpation.
2 Confirm reduction radiographically.

Caudoventral luxation

1 If the femoral head is within the obturator foramen, first release it from this position. Apply traction to the affected limb by grasping it proximal to the stifle, whilst applying counter-traction to the tuber ischium.
2 Lift the femoral head laterally and cranially into the acetabulum. This may be aided by placing a sandbag between the thighs: the sandbag then acts as a fulcrum to lever the femoral head back into the acetabulum.
3 Confirm reduction radiographically.
4 Further support following closed reduction is not required in the majority of cases.
   - **An Ehmer sling is contraindicated.**
   - Stifle hobbles may be used:
     i Create a loop out of strong adhesive tape folded on to itself, with adhesive sides together. The width of the folded adhesive tape should be sufficient for strength

and comfort. The length of the loop should be sufficient to encircle the pelvic limbs at the level of the stifles with the animal in a normal standing position.

ii   Place the loop of adhesive tape around the stifles and secure in position by wrapping further adhesive tape around the loop between the stifles.

iii   The hobble can be further secured in position with a length of tape which passes from the lateral aspect of the hobble on one side, over the dorsum of the animal, to the lateral aspect of the hobble on the other side.

Aftercare

- Exercise should be restricted for 4–6 weeks following closed reduction of hip luxation, to allow for healing of the periarticular tissues.
- Appropriate analgesia should be provided.

Potential complications

- Re-luxation of the hip
- Hip osteoarthritis
- Iatrogenic damage to the cartilage of the femoral head

FURTHER INFORMATION

Further information on hip problems and their treatment can be found in the *BSAVA Manual of Canine and Feline Musculoskeletal Disorders*.

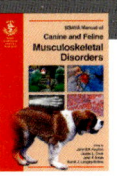

Intraosseous cannula placement

Indications/Use

- Fluid administration:
    - Where direct intravenous access is not possible (e.g. hypovolaemic puppies/kittens, severe vascular collapse), fluids normally administered intravenously can be administered via an intraosseous cannula
    - To provide *initial* fluid resuscitation and medication until intravenous access is possible

> ### WARNING
> - **Most substances that can be given intravenously can be given into the medullary space, and absorption into the vasculature is extremely rapid. However, hypertonic and alkaline fluids may cause pain and lameness.**

Contraindications

- Sites with high risk of bacterial contamination/infection, e.g. due to local tissue damage, local skin infection, diarrhoea, urinary incontinence
- Where intravenous access is possible

Equipment

- As required for **Aseptic preparation – (a) non-surgical procedures**
- Potential intraosseous cannulas:
    - Commercially available intraosseous cannulas
    - Spinal needle
    - Bone marrow aspiration needle
    - Hypodermic needle (may be able to penetrate the soft cortex of young puppies and kittens)
  Ideally, intraosseous cannulas should have a central stylet to prevent a core of bone from obstructing the cannula
  Cannula size should be appropriate for the estimated diameter of the bone marrow canal, size of the point of access into the bone and proposed fluid administration rates
- No. 11 scalpel
- Local anaesthetic
- T-connector or extension set containing heparinized saline (1 IU of heparin per ml of 0.9% saline)
- Sterile non-adherent dressing or swab
- Adhesive tape or suture
- Soft padded bandage and outer protective bandage

Patient preparation and positioning

- The animal's limb must be held still; this can usually be achieved by manual restraint but sedation may be required.

- **Aseptic preparation – (a) non-surgical procedures** should be carried out on a large area of skin surrounding the proposed site of cannula entry.
- Possible sites:
  - The medial aspect of the trochanteric fossa of the femur (see **Bone marrow aspiration**)
  - The flat medial surface of the proximal tibia, 1–2 cm distal to the tibial tuberosity
  - The cranial aspect of the greater tubercle of the humerus (see **Bone marrow aspiration**)
  - The wing of the ilium (see **Bone marrow aspiration**).

The preferred sites are those in the femur and tibia.

Technique

Tibia

1 Infiltrate local anaesthetic down to the level of the periosteum.
2 Make a stab incision in the skin over the proposed entry point into the bone.
3 Insert the cannula through the skin and directly down on to the bone.
4 Insert the cannula into the bone, using a firm twisting motion until the cannula has passed through the cortex and a small way into the medullary cavity. Entry into the medullary cavity is detected as a decrease in resistance to cannula insertion into the bone, or increased stability of the cannula within the bone. When the cannula is properly seated within the medullary cavity, movement of the cannula will result in the same movement of the bone.
5 Remove the stylet, if present.
6 Flush the cannula with heparinized saline, and attach a T-connector or infusion set.
7 Secure the cannula to the surrounding skin with sutures or tape.
8 Cover the entry site through the skin with a sterile swab or sterile non-adherent dressing.
9 Apply a bandage to the limb to protect the cannula.

Care of intraosseous cannulas

- Intraosseous cannulas are most often a short-term solution.
- Catheter patency should be maintained by any fluid running through it. If the catheter is not being used continuously, intermittent flushing with saline or heparinized saline should be performed several times a day (up to every 4 hours), as well as before and after use. If a catheter becomes blocked it should be removed.
- The bandage should be replaced and the cannula examined at least twice a day, using aseptic technique.
- The site of insertion should be monitored for signs of heat, erythema, swelling, pain or subcutaneous leakage of fluid. If these signs are noted the cannula should be removed.

- The cannula should be removed as soon as it is no longer required.

Potential complications

- Sciatic nerve damage; this can be avoided during placement of a femoral cannula, by walking the needle off the medial edge of the greater trochanter
- Growth plate damage in young animals
- Cannula displacement
- Subcutaneous leakage of fluids or medications
- Infection

Intravenous catheter placement – (a) peripheral veins

Indications/Use

- Intravenous fluid administration
- Intravenous drug administration
- Repeat intravenous blood sampling, although a central line is preferable for this indication

Contraindications

- Sites with a high risk of bacterial contamination/infection, e.g. due to local tissue damage, local skin infection, diarrhoea, urinary incontinence

Equipment

- Over-the-needle intravenous catheter, comprising a needle (or stylet) with a closely associated catheter fitted over the needle. Fluid flow rate is related to catheter length and radius. For rapid fluid administration, choose the shortest catheter with the largest radius that can pass into the vein:
    - Dogs: usually 22 G (blue), 20 G (pink) or 18 G (green)
    - Cats: usually 22 G (blue)
    - Puppies/Kittens or patients with collapsed veins may require 24 G (yellow)
- No. 11 scalpel
- T-connector or extension set containing heparinized saline (1 IU of heparin per ml of 0.9% saline), or injection cap
- Adhesive tape
- Soft padded bandage and outer protective bandage
- Appropriate skin antiseptic

> **NOTE**
>
> Sterile applicators containing 2% chlorhexidine gluconate and 70% isopropyl alcohol, designed specifically for skin antisepsis are now available. They should be used according to the manufacturer's recommendations.

Patient preparation and positioning

■ An area of skin surrounding the point of vein entry should be clipped. Long hair on the caudal aspect of the limb may need to be removed if it will interfere with securing the catheter, and to help prevent contamination. In some dogs a complete 360-degree clip of the limb may be necessary.

■ Using cotton wool or gauze swabs, the skin over the vein is prepared aseptically: see **Aseptic preparation – (a) non-surgical procedures**

■ Possible sites:
  ■ Cephalic vein and accessory cephalic vein in the distal forelimb (see **Blood sampling – (b) venous**)
  ■ Medial and lateral saphenous veins in the distal hindlimb (see **Blood sampling – (b) venous**)
  ■ Auricular veins in breeds with large ears, e.g. Basset Hound
  ■ Dorsal common digital vein of the metatarsal bones.

■ The animal's limb must be held still. This can usually be achieved by manual restraint, but sedation may be useful in animals whose temperament does not permit restraint.

Technique

ASEPSIS
Hands should be washed with an antiseptic solution prior to catheter placement. Sterile gloves are not necessary, but the precise point of catheter insertion should not be contaminated after aseptic preparation.

1 The vein is raised by an assistant placing pressure over the vein proximal to the site of catheter placement.

2 A small incision can be made in the skin over the vein but is not usually required except in dehydrated animals or those with very thick skin.

3 Advance the over-the-needle catheter through the skin into the vein, at an angle of 30–40 degrees, with the bevel of the stylet uppermost.

4 Once blood is visualized in the flash chamber of the catheter, the stylet and catheter are flattened (i.e. the angle between the catheter and the limb is reduced). Then advance the stylet/catheter unit a small distance further into the vein to ensure that the catheter lies fully within the lumen.

5 Hold the stylet in position while advancing the catheter forward off the stylet and completely into the vein.

6 Remove the stylet.

7 The assistant can now occlude the vein by applying pressure over it at the distal end of the catheter to prevent spillage of blood.

8 Connect a T-connector or extension set containing heparinized saline or an injection cap to the catheter to close it.

9 Secure the catheter firmly in place with adhesive tape, and cover with a bandage.

Care of peripheral venous catheters

- The bandage should be replaced and the catheter examined at least twice a day.
- The site of insertion should be monitored for signs of heat, erythema, swelling, pain or leakage of fluid. If signs of phlebitis are present the catheter should be removed.
- The leg and foot should be checked for swelling above the catheter site (indicating extravasation of fluid) and swelling of the toes (indicating the bandage or tape is too tight). Either of these complications necessitates catheter removal.
- Catheter patency should be maintained by any fluid running through it. If the catheter is not being used continuously, intermittent flushing with heparinized saline should be performed several times a day (up to every 4 hours) as well as before and after use. If a catheter becomes blocked it should be removed.
- When a catheter is not in use, a sterile injection cap should be used to close the catheter from the environment. Disconnection of fluid lines should be avoided and only performed when absolutely necessary to reduce contamination of the catheter.

Potential complications

- Catheter displacement/extravasation of fluids or medications
- Phlebitis/thrombophlebitis
- Thrombosis/thromboembolism
- Infection
- Dislodgement of catheter
- Air embolism
- Exsanguination

Intravenous catheter placement – (b) jugular vein (modified Seldinger technique)

Indications/Use

- Long-term (>5 days) administration of intravenous fluids
- Administration of intravenous hypertonic fluids or medications
- Repeated blood sampling
- For central venous pressure measurements
- Where maintenance of a peripheral catheter may be challenging (e.g. due to patient conformation or temperament)

Contraindications

- Coagulopathy
- Local tissue damage or skin infection in the ventral cervical region

Equipment

- As required for **Aseptic preparation – (a) non-surgical procedures**
- Sterile gloves
- Central venous Seldinger catheter pack: 4, 5 or 7 Fr double- or triple-lumen catheters would be appropriate, depending on vein diameter and length
- Over-the-needle catheter of appropriate diameter to receive the guidewire, if preferred to the introducer needle in the Seldinger pack
- No. 11 scalpel
- Heparinized saline (1 IU of heparin per ml of 0.9% saline) in two or three 5 ml syringes
- Suture materials
- Sterile dressing
- Bandaging material
- ECG monitoring equipment

Patient preparation and positioning

- Although central lines may be placed in conscious patients if they are weak or debilitated, sedation or anaesthesia is required in most animals to prevent movement during the procedure.
- Anaesthetized animals should be placed in lateral recumbency, with a sandbag positioned under the neck, and the jugular vein to be catheterized uppermost.

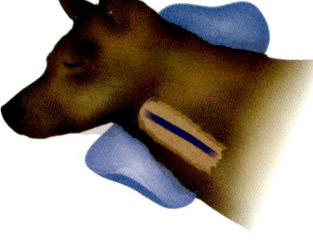

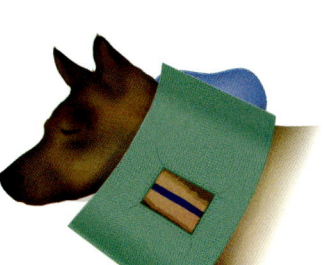

- **Aseptic preparation – (a) non-surgical procedures** is necessary, with the use of a fenestrated drape.

Technique

1 With their hand under the sterile drape, an assistant raises the jugular vein.

2 Make a 2–3 mm stab incision over the jugular vein.

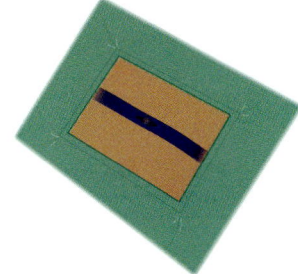

3 Insert the introducer needle or an over-the-needle catheter into the vein in a rostrocaudal direction. If using an over-the-needle catheter, then remove the needle. The assistant should then stop raising the jugular vein.

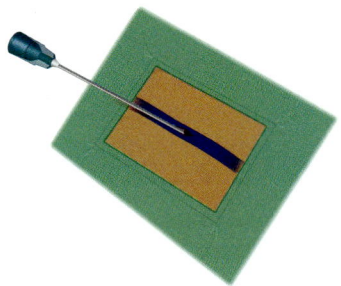

4 Insert the guidewire through the introducer needle or catheter into the jugular vein.
- The guidewire is usually held within an adapter to aid placement and may have a J-shaped tip. The J-shaped tip should be straightened by withdrawal into the adapter prior to insertion into the introducer needle or catheter.
- The ECG should be monitored for arrhythmias, as overlong wires can enter the heart.
- Care must be taken to ensure that the guidewire is held at all times for the remainder of the procedure to prevent loss of the wire into the vein.

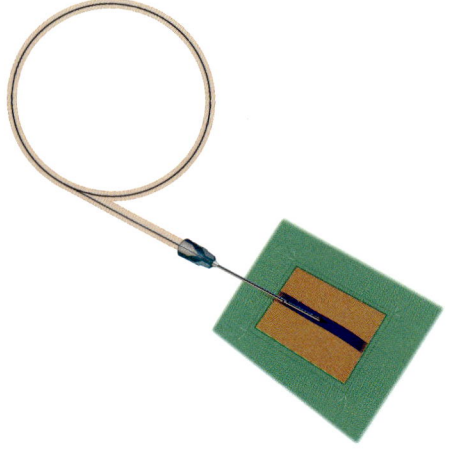

5 Remove the introducer needle or catheter, leaving the guidewire in place.

6 Advance the vessel dilator over the guidewire and into the vein to enlarge the subcutaneous tunnel; then remove the dilator.

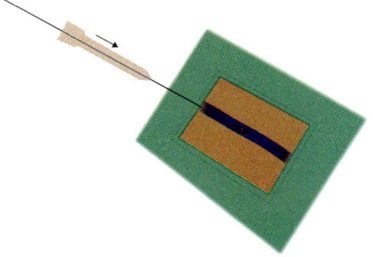

7   Advance the catheter over the wire and into the vein.

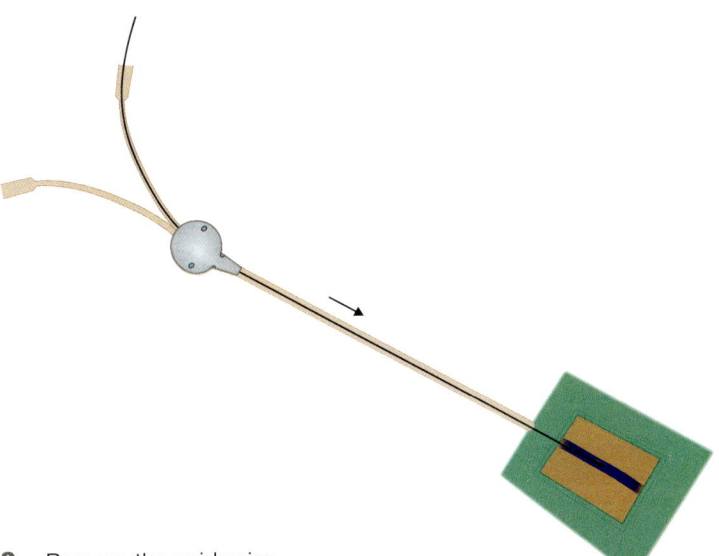

8   Remove the guidewire.

9   Place sterile injection caps, ideally incorporating on/off valves, on the end of each port of the catheter. Withdraw any air, plus some blood, from each port into a syringe part-filled with heparinized saline, to prevent air embolism and ensure intravascular placement. Then immediately flush through each port with heparinized saline. *The catheter may be prefilled with heparinized saline prior to placement, but air will enter the catheter as it is threaded over the guidewire, so this does not negate the need to check for air within the catheter after placement.*

10   Secure the catheter to the patient with sutures placed through specific suture grooves or holes in a suture wing at the base of the catheter.

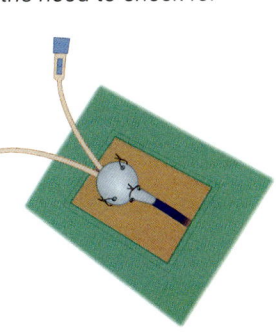

11   Place a sterile dressing over the entry site of the catheter, and bandage the catheter carefully in place. The bandage should not be too tight; it should be possible to pass a hand under it comfortably.

Care of jugular catheters

■   The bandage should be replaced and the catheter examined at least once a day. The site of insertion should be monitored for signs of heat, erythema, swelling, pain or leakage of fluid. If signs of phlebitis are present, or the animal develops unexplained pyrexia, the catheter should be removed and the tip sent for microbiological culture.

- Catheter patency should be maintained by any fluid running through it. If the catheter is not being used continuously, intermittent flushing with saline or heparinized saline (1 IU of heparin per ml of 0.9% saline) should be performed several times a day (up to every 4 hours) as well as before and after use.
- When a catheter is not in use, sterile injection caps should be used to close access ports; **ports should never be left open to the air**. Disconnection of fluid lines should be avoided, and only performed when absolutely necessary to reduce contamination of the catheter.

Potential complications

- Catheter displacement/extravasation of fluids or medications
- Phlebitis/thrombophlebitis
- Thrombosis/thromboembolism
- Infection
- Dislodgement of catheter
- Air embolism
- Exsanguination

Intravenous urography

Indications/Use

- Evaluation of renal size, shape, position and internal architecture
- Qualitative evaluation of renal function
- Demonstration of ureter position, size, integrity and patency
- Investigation of uroabdomen
- Investigation of urinary incontinence
- Investigation of haematuria or pyuria NOT arising from the lower urinary tract

Contraindications

- Renal failure
- Anuria
- Dehydration
- Hypovolaemia
- Known or suspected hypersensitivity to iodinated contrast media

Equipment

- As required for **Urethral catheterization** and **Intravenous catheter placement – (a) peripheral veins**
- Water-soluble contrast medium for intravenous use (see below for concentrations and dose rates) (see also **Iodinated contrast media**)
- 20–50 ml syringe
- Giving set
- 500 ml bag of 0.9% saline

Patient preparation and positioning

- In an elective examination, withhold food *from 24 hours before* the procedure.
- Give at least one non-irritant cleansing enema (e.g. warm water) *2–3 hours prior* to examination.
- The procedure should be performed under general anaesthesia, since injection of contrast medium in the conscious patient may cause retching, vomiting and struggling. Moreover, should an idiosyncratic reaction/anaphylaxis to contract media occur, airway patency can be maintained.
- Pass a urinary catheter and drain the bladder of urine (see **Urethral catheterization**). The catheter can be left *in situ* but should be pulled out of the bladder and into the proximal urethra.
- Positioning will be determined by views required (see below).

Technique

There are two basic techniques:

- High-concentration, low-volume (bolus) IVU, with or without abdominal compression: preferred for imaging the kidneys
- Low-concentration, high-volume (infusion) IVU: preferred for imaging the ureters. This technique may produce inferior renal opacification but gives improved visibility of the ureters due to increased osmotic diuresis. This technique also has less strict requirements for the timing of radiographs.

High-concentration, low-volume (bolus) IVU:

1 Obtain lateral and ventrodorsal plain radiographs of the abdomen to check exposure factors and to allow comparison with subsequent contrast images.
2 Plain radiographs should also be used to assess adequate patient preparation. If this appears to be incomplete, repeated warm water enemas ± digital evacuation should be performed.
3 Position the patient in dorsal recumbency, as the ventrodorsal view is more helpful initially.
4 Inject contrast medium at room temperature or warmed to 37°C (to reduce viscosity) at 300–400 mg iodine/ml (concentration is given as a number after the trade name) rapidly into a cephalic vein via a catheter. Dose rate is 800 mg iodine/kg bodyweight (i.e. about 2 ml/kg).
5 Immediately take the first radiograph.
6 Take further ventrodorsal radiographs at regular intervals (e.g. 2, 5, 10 and 15 minutes) until a clear nephrogram and pyelogram are obtained. Then obtain a lateral view ± oblique views to visualize the ureters.
7 Continue until a diagnosis is made or a normal appearance is confirmed.

Low-concentration, high-volume (infusion) IVU:

1 Obtain lateral and ventrodorsal plain radiographs to check exposure factors and to allow comparison with subsequent

contrast images. If the study is to demonstrate the location of the ureter endings in incontinent patients, a pneumocystogram should be obtained to outline the bladder neck.

2 Administer contrast medium at room temperature or warmed to 37°C (to reduce viscosity) at 150 mg iodine/ml (more concentrated media can be diluted with 0.9% saline) over 5–30 minutes into the cephalic vein via a catheter. Dose rate is 1200 mg iodine/kg bodyweight (i.e. 8 ml/kg).

3 Obtain radiographs as above, starting approximately 5 minutes into the infusion until a diagnosis is made, or a normal appearance is confirmed.

Potential complications

- Idiosyncratic reaction/anaphylaxis (rare): risk proportional to speed of injection, concentration of agent and volume infused
- Renal failure (rare): more likely with pre-existing renal disease; therefore, ensure adequate hydration before and during the procedure

> **FURTHER INFORMATION**
>
> Further details of these procedures and their interpretation can be found in the *BSAVA Manual of Canine and Feline Abdominal Imaging* and the *BSAVA Manual of Canine and Feline Nephrology and Urology*.
>
>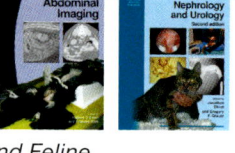

Iodinated contrast media

Iodinated contrast media appear radiopaque on a radiograph due to iodine having a higher atomic number than soft tissues. There is a wide range of iodinated contrast media available. None is authorized for veterinary use and most are POM.

Constituent	Properties	Trade name	Uses			Formulations (mg iodine/ml)
			Spinal	Vascular, urinary	GI	
Iothalamate meglumine	Monomer Ionic High-osmolar	Conray	–	+	–	141; 202; 282; 400
Sodium meglumine diatrizoate	Monomer Ionic High-osmolar	Urografin	–	+	–	146; 325; 370
Iohexol	Monomer Non-ionic Low-osmolar	Omnipaque	+	+	+	140; 240; 300; 350

Use

- Contrast studies of the GI and urinary tracts (see **Intravenous urography, Retrograde urethrography/vaginourethrography**), angiography, arthrography, sialography, dacryocystography, sino- or fistulography, and myelography
- Only non-ionic agents may be used for myelography, but not all non-ionic agents are authorized for myelography in humans
- Fluid and electrolyte disturbances should be corrected prior to use

Contraindications

- Known or suspected hypersensitivity to iodinated contrast media
- Should be used with care in animals with moderate to severe renal impairment. Iodinated contrast media are primarily excreted via the kidneys, and pre-existing renal disease predisposes to contrast media-induced renal failure
- Anuria
- Dehydration
- Hypovolaemia

Adverse reactions

- More common with ionic than non-ionic media and with hyperosmolar media:
    - Anaphylaxis may occur following i.v. injection of any iodinated contrast medium
    - Nausea, vomiting, hypotension, dyspnoea, erythema, urticaria, sensation of heat, and cardiac rate or rhythm disturbances have been reported in humans following i.v. injection
    - Seizures or transient motor or sensory dysfunction have been reported in humans following myelography
    - Aspiration of high osmolar contrast medium may result in pulmonary oedema
    - May aggravate clinical signs in patients with myasthenia gravis
- Non-ionic low-osmolar and iso-osmolar agents have fewer adverse effects on the cardiovascular system and are safer in neonates and animals with cardiovascular disease
- When used intravascularly, catheters should be flushed regularly to minimize risk of clotting; non-ionic media have less anticoagulant activity *in vitro* than ionic preparations
- Extravasation of high-osmolar agents may rarely lead to soft tissue injury
- Warming the contrast medium prior to injection reduces minor side effects

Drug interactions

- Iodinated contrast media decrease thyroid uptake of iodine and preclude therapeutic radioiodine therapy for 2 months following administration
- Hypersensitivity reactions may be aggravated in patients on beta-blocker medication

Local anaesthesia – nerve blocks

Indications/Use

- Treatment of perioperative pain, in conjunction with heavy sedation or general anaesthesia
- Local anaesthesia as part of a multimodal approach to analgesia
- *Specific indications for each block are listed under each technique*

Contraindications

- Infection (including pyoderma) or neoplasia that might be disseminated by the passage of the needle
- Septicaemia, bleeding disorders, hypovolaemia, hypotension and altered neurological function for epidural anaesthesia and analgesia

Equipment

- Local anaesthetics:

Drug	Onset time (minutes)	Duration of action (hours)	Recommended doses in healthy animals (mg/kg)	Toxic dose (mg/kg)
Lidocaine	5–15	1–2	Dogs: 4–6 Cats: 2	Dogs: 10 Cats: 4
Bupivacaine	20–30	2.5–6	Dogs: 2 Cats: 1.5	Dogs: 4 Cats: 2
Ropivacaine	2–20	2–6	Dogs: 1.5	Dogs: 4

> **NOTES**
>
> - Bupivacaine and ropivacaine are not authorized for use in dogs and cats in the UK.
> - The toxic doses listed above are conservative estimates, to minimize the occurrence of toxicity.
> - Local anaesthetic doses are most often based on the space available around nerves and so are given as volumes in technique descriptions; however, volume recommendations should always be checked against recommended mg/kg doses.
> - Preservative-free solutions are required for epidural use.
> - Preservative-free morphine (0.1–0.2mg/kg) can be used for epidural analgesia.

- Range of needles: $3/8$ to 1 inch; 21, 23 G
- Range of spinal needles: 1.5, 2.5, 3.5 inch; 20, 22 G
- Range of syringes: 1–20 ml
- Loss-of-resistance syringes for epidural technique are available in 5 ml, 8 ml and 10 ml

- Ultrasound machine or nerve stimulator locator: these can be used to locate the nerves and aid accurate needle placement and thus the effectiveness of the nerve block. They are absolutely recommended for the paravertebral brachial plexus block

Patient preparation and positioning

- Sedation or anaesthesia permits easier positioning of animals, identification of anatomical landmarks, isolation of specific nerves and blood vessels, and more precise/less traumatic needle placement.
- **Aseptic preparation – (a) non-surgical procedures** must be performed at the proposed site of needle insertion.

Technique

> **WARNING**
>
> - **The aim is to inject local anaesthetic around a nerve:**
>   - **After needle insertion, but prior to injection of local anaesthetic, *always* aspirate to check for blood to avoid intravenous or arterial injection of local anaesthetic**
>   - **If a high pressure (more than experienced with a normal intramuscular injection) is felt on injection of the local anaesthetic, the needle may be within the nerve; withdraw the needle and start again to avoid nerve damage.**

Head

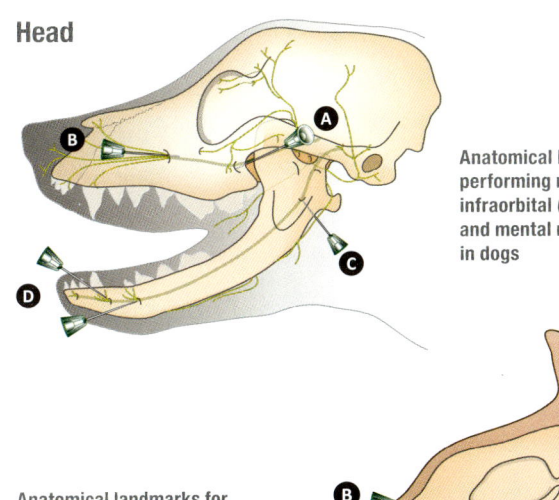

Anatomical landmarks for performing maxillary (A), infraorbital (B), mandibular (C) and mental nerve blocks (D) in dogs

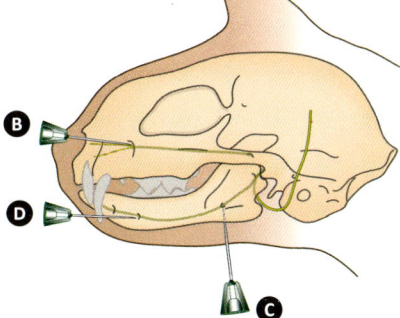

Anatomical landmarks for performing infraorbital (B), mandibular (C) and mental nerve blocks (D) in cats

Infraorbital nerve block

- Desensitizes the upper lip, nose and skin rostroventral to the infraorbital foramen.
- Position animal in lateral recumbency.

Dogs:
1. Palpate the infraorbital foramen on the lateral surface of the maxilla – intraorally by lifting the upper lip, or percutaneously.
2. Direct a 25 G needle in a caudal direction, parallel to the infraorbital canal, a short distance into the infraorbital foramen.
3. Elevate the dog's nose and occlude the entrance to the infraorbital foramen with light finger pressure.
4. Inject 0.1–1.0 ml of local anaesthetic solution caudally into the infraorbital canal.

Cats:
1. Palpate the ridge of bone overlying the infraorbital foramen; the foramen cannot be palpated directly.
2. Insert a 25 G needle intraorally or percutaneously, dorsal and parallel to the premolar teeth, in a caudal direction towards the infraorbital ridge.
3. Inject a maximum of 0.3 ml of local anaesthetic solution directly on to the infraorbital nerve.

Maxillary nerve block

- Desensitizes the hard and soft palate, upper teeth and gingiva, nose, and the skin over the maxilla.
- Position animal in lateral recumbency.

1. Palpate the rostral end of the zygomatic arch where it meets the maxilla.
2. Insert a 21–25 G needle percutaneously just ventral to this point, and direct the needle in a vertical direction perpendicular to the sagittal plane.
3. Inject 0.1–1.5 ml (dogs) or 0.1–0.3 ml (cats) of local anaesthetic solution directly on to the maxillary nerve.

Mental nerve block

- Desensitizes the lower lip and chin rostral to the injection site.
- Position animal in lateral recumbency.

1. Palpate the middle mental foramen intraorally, on the lateral surface of the rostral mandible: adjacent to the 2nd premolar tooth in **dogs;** or just rostral to the premolar teeth in **cats**.
2. Direct a 21–25 G needle rostrocaudally, just inside the foramen.
3. Inject 0.1–1.5 ml (dogs) or 0.1–0.3 ml (cats) of local anaesthetic solution caudally into the foramen.

Mandibular nerve block

- Desensitizes the lower teeth, gingiva, tongue and chin.
- Position animal in lateral recumbency.

1 Palpate the mandibular foramen on the medial surface of the mandible just rostral to the angular process.

2 Insert a 22–25 G needle percutaneously along the ventral border of the mandible, ventral to the mandibular foramen.

3 Direct the needle rostrally along the medial border of the mandible towards the mandibular foramen.

4 Inject 0.2–1.0 ml (dogs) or 0.1–0.3 ml (cats) of local anaesthetic solution directly on to the mandibular nerve as it enters the mandibular foramen.

Auriculotemporal and great auricular nerve block (dog)

■ Desensitizes the inner surface of the auricular cartilage and the external ear canal.

■ Position the dog in lateral recumbency.

1 Palpate the 'V' formed by the caudal aspect of the zygomatic arch and vertical ear canal.

2 Insert a 21–25 G needle percutaneously, directing it towards the point of this 'V'.

3 Inject 0.1–0.5 ml of local anaesthetic.

4 Palpate the wing of the atlas vertebra.

5 Insert a 21–25 G needle percutaneously, ventral to the wing of atlas, and direct the needle parallel and adjacent to the vertical ear canal.

6 Inject 0.5–1.0 ml of local anaesthetic solution.

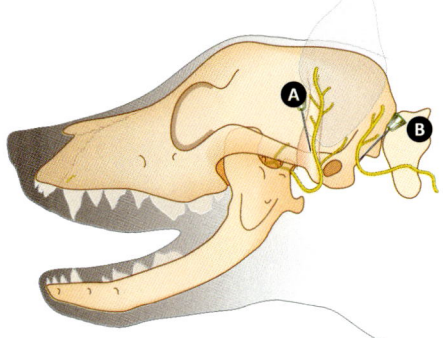

Anatomical landmarks for performing auriculotemporal (A) and great auricular (B) nerve blocks in dogs

Limb

Paravertebral brachial plexus block (dog)

■ Desensitizes the entire forelimb.

■ Position the dog in lateral recumbency. An assistant can elevate the scapula away from the thorax to aid access to the caudal cervical vertebrae and first rib.

1 Palpate the transverse process of C6.

2 Insert a 22 G, 1.5–3 inch spinal needle percutaneously, and direct it towards the cranial and caudal margins of the transverse process of C6 to access the ventral branches of spinal nerves C6 and C7. The needle should be angled caudally to avoid intrapleural penetration.

3 Inject 1–3 ml of local anaesthetic solution around each nerve.

4 Palpate the head of the first rib.

5 Insert the needle percutaneously and direct it toward the cranial and ventral borders of the dorsal part of the first rib to access spinal nerves C8 and T1.

6 Inject 1–3 ml of local anaesthetic solution around each nerve.

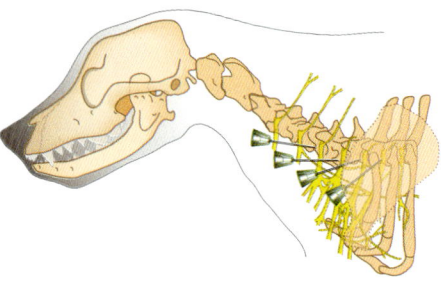

Anatomical landmarks for performing paravertebral blockade of the brachial plexus in dogs (dotted line shows normal anatomical position of the scapula)

Axillary brachial plexus block

- Desensitizes the forelimb below the level of the elbow; excludes the shoulder and humerus.
- Position animal in lateral recumbency.

1 Insert a 22 G, 1 inch needle (**cats**) or 22 G, 1.5–3 inch spinal needle (**dogs**) percutaneously into the axillary space at the level of the shoulder, and direct it towards the first rib.

2 Inject local anaesthetic: 10–15 ml is required for a 25 kg dog; 1 ml is sufficient for a cat.

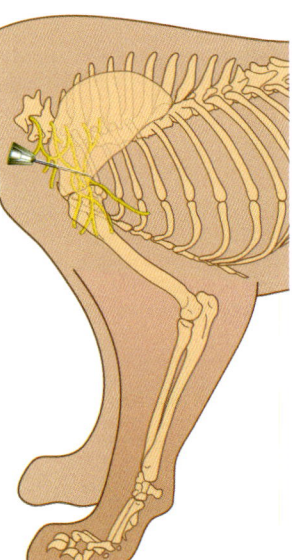

Anatomical landmarks for performing axillary blockade of the brachial plexus in cats

Radial, ulnar, median and musculocutaneous nerve blocks

- Desensitizes the forepaw in **cats;** and the forelimb distal to the elbow in **dogs**.
- Position animal in lateral recumbency with the affected limb uppermost.

Dogs:

1 Palpate the lateral and medial humeral condyles.

2 Insert a 22 G, 1 inch needle percutaneously, proximal to the lateral epicondyle of the humerus.

3 Direct the needle between the brachialis muscle and lateral head of the triceps to access the radial nerve.

4 Inject 1–3 ml of local anaesthetic solution directly on to the nerve.

5 Direct the needle percutaneously, proximal to the medial epicondyle of the humerus, and between the biceps brachii muscle and medial head of the triceps to access the ulnar, median and musculocutaneous nerves.

6 Inject 1–3 ml of local anaesthetic solution into the space surrounding these three nerves.

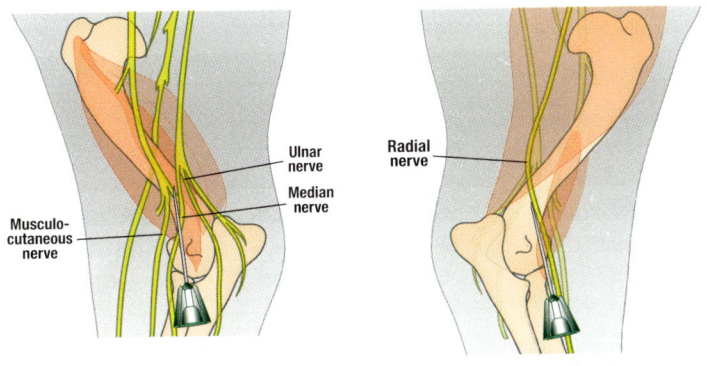

Anatomical landmarks for performing radial, ulnar, median and musculocutaneous nerve blocks in dogs

Cats:

1 Grasp the forepaw.

2 Insert a 25 G, $^3/_8$ to 1 inch needle and pass it subcutaneously just proximal to the carpus along the dorsomedial border of the distal antebrachium to access the radial nerve.

3 Inject 0.1 ml of local anaesthetic solution.

4 Pass the needle subcutaneously, medial and lateral to the accessory pad on the palmar surface of the paw to access the medial and ulnar nerves.

5 Inject 0.1 ml of local anaesthetic solution per nerve.

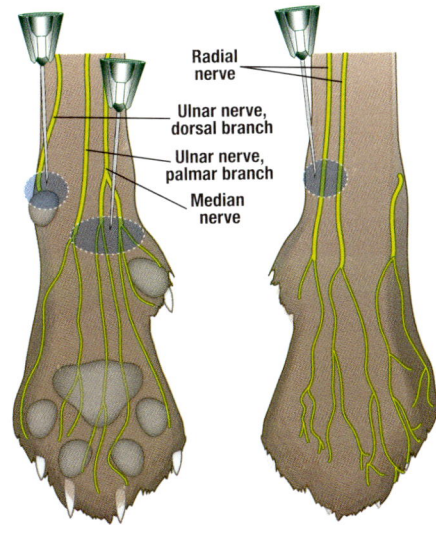

Anatomical landmarks for performing nerve blocks of the distal branches of the radial, ulnar and median nerves in cats. Shaded areas within dotted lines show areas to be blocked

Saphenous, common peroneal and tibial nerve blocks

- Desensitizes the pelvic limb distal to the stifle.
- Position animal in lateral recumbency with the affected limb uppermost.
- A 22–25 G, $^3/_8$ to 1 inch needle is used.
- 1–3 ml (**dogs**) or 0.1–0.3 ml (**cats**) of local anaesthetic solution is injected directly on to each nerve.

The *saphenous nerve* runs through the femoral triangle on the medial surface of the thigh. The nerve lies cranial to the femoral artery and vein. The needle is inserted percutaneously directly over the nerve cranial to the pulsations of the femoral artery.

The *common peroneal nerve* runs laterally over the gastrocnemius muscle and across the lateral surface of the fibular head. The nerve is palpated distal to the fibular head: the needle is inserted percutaneously, directly over the nerve.

The *tibial nerve* runs deep to the medial and lateral heads of the gastrocnemius muscle, and then between the tendons of the superficial digital flexor and long digital extensor. The needle can be inserted next to the nerve at either of these locations.

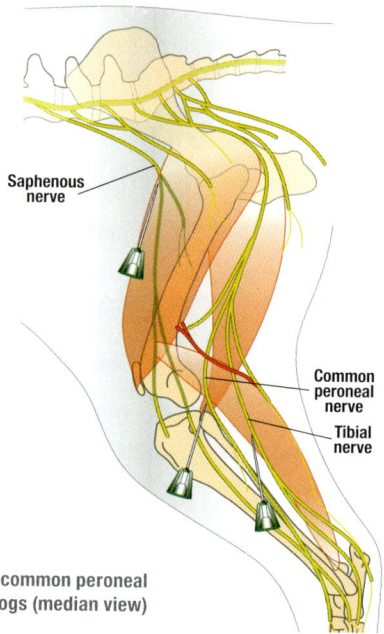

Anatomical landmarks for saphenous, common peroneal and tibial nerve blocks in dogs (median view)

Epidural anaesthesia and analgesia

- Provides perioperative analgesia for surgery of the pelvis, pelvic limbs and perineal region, and is used in combination with general anaesthesia to reduce anaesthetic requirements and to improve analgesia and muscle relaxation.
- Position animal in sternal recumbency. The animal should be positioned squarely on the table with the pelvic limbs pulled cranially to lie alongside the abdomen.

> **NOTE**
>
> Preservative-free solutions must be used for epidural injection.

1 Palpate the indentation overlying the lumbosacral junction. This is positioned caudal to a line drawn between the left and right iliac crests, and lies along the midline between the dorsal spinous process of the 7th lumbar vertebra and the median sacral crest.

2 Insert a 20 G (dog) or 22 G (cat), 1.5–2.5 inch spinal needle percutaneously along the dorsal midline, perpendicular to the skin and directed towards the lumbosacral space.

3 Advance the needle gently. An increase in resistance followed by an abrupt loss of resistance or 'pop' is encountered as the needle passes through the ligamentum flavum and enters the epidural space. Stop advancing the needle once the epidural space has been entered. Stabilize the needle with one hand and remove the stylet with the other.

4 If CSF is noted in the hub of the needle (possible in a cat due to extension of the spinal cord and meninges into the lumbosacral space) withdraw the needle slightly into the epidural space. If blood is noted in the hub of the needle, replace the stylet and reposition the needle.

5 A loss-of-resistance syringe containing 0.5 ml (**cat**) or 1 ml (**dog**) of air is attached to the needle. Lack of resistance to injection of air indicates correct needle placement.

6 Draw preservative-free local anaesthetic solution into a syringe:
- **Dogs:** 1 ml/6 kg for desensitization of the pelvic limbs, or 1 ml/4 kg for desensitization to the level of the umbilicus to a maximum of 6 ml
- **Cats:** 1 ml/5 kg.

7 Draw an additional 0.5–1 ml of air into the syringe.

8 Attach the syringe to the needle. Inject local anaesthetic slowly over at least 30 seconds. Collapse of the air in the syringe indicates an increase in resistance and that the tip of the needle is no longer in the epidural space.

ALTERNATIVES

- An alternative technique for checking the correct position of the needle in the epidural space can be used. The stylet of the needle is removed following skin penetration and a drop of 0.9% sterile saline is dropped into the hub of the needle. Advancement of the needle into the epidural space results in suction of saline from the hub into the needle. This avoids the possible complication of air embolism.
- In addition to, or instead of local anaesthetics, 0.1–0.2 mg/kg preservative-free morphine can be used. This provides perioperative analgesia for pelvic limb, perineal, abdominal and thoracic procedures for 12–24 hours.

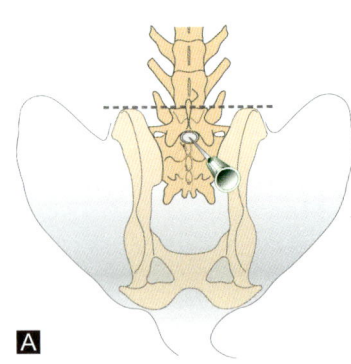

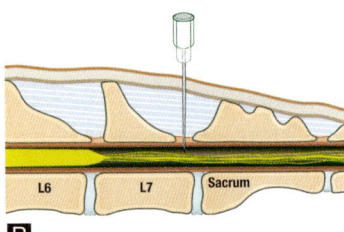

B

Anatomical landmarks for performing lumbosacral epidural anaesthesia and analgesia in dogs. The lumbosacral space can be found caudal to a line drawn between the cranial borders of the ilia (marked with a dotted line). **A** Dorsal view. **B** Lateral view.

Complications

- Nerve damage due to direct injection *into* a nerve
- Systemic toxicity due to overdose of local anaesthetic or direct injection of local anaesthetic into a blood vessel. CNS toxicity results in depression, seizures, muscle tremors and respiratory depression. Cardiac toxicity results in hypotension, arrhythmias and cardiac arrest
- Local tissue irritation and nerve damage
- Allergic reactions to the local anaesthetic or to preservative agents in proprietary preparations
- Brachial plexus blocks can be associated with pneumothorax, Horner's syndrome, epidural injection and compromise to respiratory function due to phrenic nerve block. However, unilateral phrenic nerve block is usually well tolerated.
- Epidural anaesthesia using non-toxic doses of local anaesthetics can be associated with significant peripheral vasodilation, hypotension, respiratory depression and Horner's syndrome. These complications are more likely with high volumes of local anaesthetic agents
- Epidural anaesthesia with opioids can be associated with urinary retention for up to 24 hours
- Epidural anaesthesia in the cat can be associated with intrathecal injection or direct injury to the spinal cord
- Air embolism is a complication of air injection into the epidural space

---

FURTHER INFORMATION

For details of anaesthetic and analgesic protocols see the *BSAVA Manual of Canine and Feline Anaesthesia and Analgesia.*

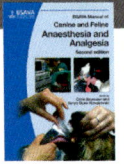

Myringotomy

Indications/Use

- To obtain samples for diagnostic evaluation of otitis media
- To permit lavage of the tympanic bulla for non-surgical management of otitis media

Contraindications

- Otitis externa, as there is a risk of transfer of disease to the middle ear

Equipment

- Otoscope with a sterilized otoscopic speculum; a video-otoscope is best but not essential
- Sterile catheters (e.g. 3.5 Fr tomcat catheter or long polypropylene catheter) of sufficient length to access the tympanic membrane via the working channel of a video-otoscope, or along the speculum of an ordinary otoscope
- 2.5 or 5 ml, plus two 20 ml syringes
- 3-way tap
- Sterile saline
- Otic ceruminolytic agent (may be needed in dogs)
- Bacteriological swab
- EDTA sample pots
- Microscope slides

Patient preparation and positioning

- In chronic otitis externa, a short course of systemic glucocorticoids may aid optimal visualization of the tympanic membrane.
- General anaesthesia is required.
- A properly placed and inflated endotracheal tube is recommended due to possible drainage of fluid from the middle ear canal into the pharynx.
- The animal is placed in lateral or sternal recumbency. A towel may be used to elevate the caudal head and neck slightly in relation to the muzzle.
- The animal's eyes should be protected if ceruminolytics are used to clean the external ear canal.

Technique

> **HEALTH AND SAFETY**
>
> Personnel should wear gloves, face mask and, ideally, eye protectors to avoid contact with contaminated aerosols.

1 Clean and dry the external ear canal.
- Cleaning can be performed safely with sterile saline.
- Ceruminolytic agents can be used in dogs to speed removal of waxy exudates, but must be flushed completely from the ear canal with sterile saline.

- Ceruminolytics should **not** be used to flush the ears of cats if the integrity of the tympanic membrane is uncertain, due to the higher risk of neurological complications.
- Drying can be achieved by suction of lavage solutions.

2   Insert the otoscope into the external ear canal to visualize the tympanic membrane. This requires straightening of the external ear canal, by pulling the pinna dorsally and outwards away from the head.

3   Under direct visualization, flush the ear canal with sterile saline to remove any remaining debris.
- A long polypropylene catheter attached to a 3-way tap and two 20 ml syringes can achieve efficient flushing and suction.
- The person controlling the otoscope visualizes and positions the tip of the catheter, while an assistant flushes in saline with one syringe and removes the fluid by suction through the second syringe.

4   The site of myringotomy should be ventral. Position the otoscope carefully to visualize this site.

5   Cut the tip of the catheter at an angle to make it sharp enough to incise the tympanic membrane.

6   Under direct visualization, pass the tip of the catheter through the ventral aspect of the tympanic membrane into the middle ear and maintain it in this position.

7   An assistant should infuse 1 ml of sterile saline via the catheter into the middle ear, and then aspirate to obtain a fluid sample for cytology and culture.

8   The assistant should then flush the middle ear gently with sterile saline until the fluid aspirated back is clear.

9   Remove the catheter from the middle ear.

10 Remove the otoscope.

Potential complications

- Neurological signs (including head shaking, Horner's syndrome, deafness) can result from over-aggressive lavage or the use of ceruminolytics

> **FURTHER INFORMATION**
>
> This technique is illustrated in the *BSAVA Manual of Canine and Feline Endoscopy and Endosurgery*; cytological findings are discussed in the *BSAVA Manual of Canine and Feline Clinical Pathology*.

Nasal oxygen administration

Indications/Use

- Patients requiring oxygen for several days
- Patients that do not tolerate an oxygen mask
- Patients that are too large to fit inside an oxygen cage

Contraindications

- Inspired oxygen concentrations may not be high enough for very hypoxic animals, particularly if they are mouth-breathing. In very hypoxic animals, bilateral nasal oxygen lines can be used
- Not useful for brachycephalic animals or patients with facial disease or pain

Equipment

- Rubber catheter/soft polythene feeding tube (large dogs: 5–10 Fr, depending on the size of the animal; 5 Fr in cats and dogs <5 kg) or nasal prongs
- Topical local anaesthetic (e.g. 0.5% proxymetacaine eyedrops)
- Sterile aqueous lubricant (e.g. K-Y jelly)
- Non-absorbable suture material, needle and needle-holders
- Tissue glue
- 25 mm wide adhesive tape
- Oxygen delivery system
- Humidifier (container filled with distilled water)
- Elizabethan collar

Patient preparation and positioning

- Usually performed in the conscious animal, although fractious animals may benefit from light sedation.
- The patient is positioned in sternal recumbency, or sitting.
- Apply several drops of local anaesthetic down one nostril and wait approximately 10 minutes before inserting the catheter.

Technique

Nasal catheter

1   Measure the distance from the nares to the medial canthus of the eye and mark this on the catheter.
2   Following desensitization of the nostril with topical local anaesthetic, gently insert the lubricated catheter into the nostril in a ventromedial direction (toward the base of the opposite ear) and advance it to the pre-determined mark. The nasal planum can be pushed dorsally to direct the tube ventrally.
3   Once the catheter is in place, it is contoured around the alar fold, and sutured or glued in place on the side of the face. For the most secure placement, a suture should be placed as close to the nasal-cutaneous junction as possible.

4   Attach the nasal catheter to an oxygen delivery system with flow rates of 100–200 ml/kg/minute.
5   Humidify the oxygen by bubbling it through a chamber filled with distilled water.
6   Place an Elizabethan collar.

Nasal prongs

- Some animals can be best managed using bilateral nasal 'prongs' that penetrate 1 cm or less into the nasal cavity.
- Inspired oxygen concentrations of 30–50% can easily be achieved using this type of system, although panting probably limits their effectiveness.

Potential complications

- Long-term therapy with high concentrations of oxygen (F_iO_2 >0.6 for >12 hours, or sooner with assisted ventilation) can be associated with lung damage ('oxygen toxicity'). Although rare, every effort should be made to minimize F_iO_2 for critically ill patients
- Sneezing and dislodgement of catheter or prongs
- Nasal discharge is common but is not clinically significant

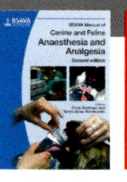
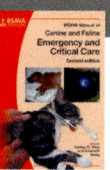

FURTHER INFORMATION

Further information on administration of supplementary oxygen, including the use of masks and oxygen cages, can be found in the *BSAVA Manual of Canine and Feline Anaesthesia and Analgesia* and the *BSAVA Manual of Canine and Feline Emergency and Critical Care*.

Naso-oesophageal tube placement

Indications/Use

- Short-term nutritional support (up to 7 days) of cats or small dogs. In medium to large dogs, the sheer volume of a liquid diet required to meet the energy needs generally limits the usefulness of this feeding method
- Animals that require assisted feeding but in which general anaesthesia is contraindicated

Contraindications

- Comatose, recumbent or dysphoric animals at risk of aspiration
- Head trauma

- Nasopharyngeal disease
- Persistent vomiting
- Absent gag reflex
- Severe nasal disease or dysphagia
- Oesophagitis or severe oesophageal dysfunction
  (e.g. megaoesophagus)

Equipment

- Naso-oesophageal tube (soft polyvinyl or silicone)
  - Cats: 3–5 Fr; 40–75 cm
  - Dogs: 4–8 Fr; 40–80 cm
- 5–10 ml syringe
- 5 ml syringe containing sterile water for injection
- Topical local anaesthetic drops, e.g. proxymetacaine 0.5%
- Lubricating jelly, e.g. K–Y jelly
- Permanent marker pen
- 25 mm wide adhesive tape
- Tissue glue
- Elizabethan collar

Patient preparation and positioning

- The procedure is normally performed with gentle minimal restraint.
- Occasionally light sedation may be required.
- The patient can be positioned standing, or in lateral or sternal recumbency.
- The animal's head should be restrained and slightly raised.

Technique

1   Instil local anaesthetic drops into one nostril, and allow at least 2 minutes to take effect. Either nostril can be used, but if you are right-handed it is generally easier to place the tube into the animal's left nostril.
2   Measure the distance from the nose to the 9th rib and mark this on the tube with a permanent marker pen. Alternatively, place a piece of tape 1 cm distal to this point.
3   Lubricate the first centimetre of the tube to aid insertion.
4   Insert the tube gently (but initially rapidly for the first 3–4 cm to avoid it being sneezed out), aiming ventromedially (toward the base of the opposite ear) so that it will pass into the ventral meatus of the nasal cavity. The nasal planum can be pushed dorsally to direct the tube ventrally.
5   Insert the remainder of the tube slowly until it reaches the marked predetermined position (nose to 9th rib). Watch for signs of swallowing (indicating the tube is correctly in the oesophagus) and coughing or discomfort (indicating the tube may have been inserted into the trachea). In the latter case, the tube should be removed and repositioned.

6 Check that the tube is positioned correctly by performing at least two of the following three procedures:

    a Attach an empty 5–10 ml syringe and apply suction:

- If the tube is in the trachea, syringefuls of air will be readily withdrawn. If this occurs the tube should be removed
- If suction creates a vacuum, meaning that no air can be sucked into the tube, it should be in the oesophagus

    b Attach a syringe containing the 5 ml of sterile water for injection and slowly flush it down the tube, watching for coughing and/or restlessness. If these signs occur, stop flushing and remove the tube

    c Inject 5–10 ml of air whilst auscultating the left abdomen. If borborygmus is heard, the tube is correctly placed.

> **NOTE**
>
> Tube placement should be reassessed using these methods prior to administration of each feed.

7 A lateral thoracic radiograph should also be taken to confirm: that the tube is in the correct position; where the end lies (distal third of the oesophagus, not the stomach); and that the tube is not kinked or twisted.

8 Place two butterfly tape strips on the tube, approximately 1 and 3 cm from the nostril. Apply a thin layer of glue to each strip; bend the tube up and around the dorsal aspect of the animal's nose and head, and press it on to the hair. *Alternatively,* in larger breeds of dog, especially those with long muzzles, the tube may be best positioned along the ipsilateral muzzle and below the ipsilateral ear.

9 Place an Elizabethan collar to prevent the animal displacing the tube. The remaining length of tube can be coiled and taped inside the collar.

10 Feeding can commence immediately after tube placement.

Feeding

> **NOTES**
>
> - As the feeding tubes are of narrow bore, a liquid diet must be used.
> - *Before* feeding each time, check the position of the tube as detailed in Step 6 above. Radiographs should be taken if there is any doubt about the position of the tube.

1 Flush the tube with small amounts (5–10 ml) of lukewarm tap water.

2 Food should be warmed to body temperature and injected into the tube over approximately 5 minutes.

- Feed only one third of the resting energy requirement (RER) on the first day.

- On the second day, feed two-thirds of the RER, increasing to the entire RER on day three.
- Divide the daily requirement into multiple (5 or 6) feeds per 24 hours.

3 Flush the tube *after* every feed with 5–10 ml of lukewarm tap water.

RER

The resting energy requirement is now used as the 'baseline' energy recommendation for hospitalized dogs and cats, regardless of the disease or surgery.

The following equation can be used to calculate the RER in kcal/day for cats or dogs:

$$RER = 70 \times bodyweight\ (kg)^{0.75}$$

Alternatively, for animals >2 kg the following equation can be used:

$$RER = 30 \times bodyweight\ (kg) + 70$$

Note: To convert kcal to kilojoules (kJ) multiply by 4.185

Tube maintenance and removal

- Twice a day, the external nares should be wiped gently with cotton wool soaked in water.
- If the tube becomes blocked, 3 ml of a carbonated drink (e.g. cola or soda water) can be instilled and left for 5–10 minutes to help dislodge blockages.
- The tube can be removed at any time following placement. The hair under the butterfly tape strips should be gently cut and the tube removed in one motion. Light sedation may be required in non-cooperative patients.

Potential complications

- Rhinitis
- Vomiting
- Regurgitation
- Aspiration pneumonia
- Tube dislodgement or removal

FURTHER INFORMATION

Further details on assisted feeding can be found in the *BSAVA Manual of Canine and Feline Rehabilitation, Supportive and Palliative Care*.

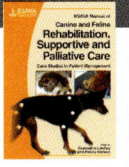

Oesophagostomy tube placement

Indications/Use

- Nutritional support for weeks to months

Contraindications

- Comatose, recumbent or dysphoric animals at risk of aspiration
- Persistent vomiting – the tube may be expelled or retroflexed into the nasopharynx
- Oesophagitis or severe oesophageal dysfunction (e.g. megaoesophagus)

Equipment

- As required for **Aseptic preparation – (a) surgical procedures**
- Oesophagostomy tube (open-end, silicone with multiple side holes or red rubber feeding tube) for surgical cut-down technique:
  - Cats: 10–14 Fr; 23-38 cm long
  - Dogs: 14–19 Fr; 38 cm long
- OR a percutaneous oesophagostomy tube placement kit (containing oesophagostomy tube, rigid introducer and needle with peel-away sheath):
  - 10 G, 5 cm long needle and peel-away sheath; use with 10 Fr catheter (cats)
  - 8 G, 7 cm long needle and peel-away sheath; use with 12 Fr catheter (cats and small dogs)
  - 7 G, 7 cm long needle and peel-away sheath; use with 14 Fr catheter (medium and large dogs)
- Long curved forceps (minimum 20cm), e.g. Rochester–Carmalt
- Scalpel blade
- Laryngoscope
- 25 mm wide adhesive tape
- Suture material, e.g. 3 metric (2/0 USP) monofilament nylon
- Sterile dressing to cover the tube site
- Materials for a soft, padded, loose, neck bandage
- Permanent marker pen

Patient preparation and positioning

- General anaesthesia is required.
- The patient is placed in right lateral recumbency.
- **Aseptic preparation – (a) surgical procedures** is required from the dorsal to the ventral aspects of the neck and from the angle of the jaw to the shoulder.

Technique

Two methods are available.

Surgical cut-down

Photos courtesy of David Walker, Anderson Moores Veterinary Specialists

1 An assistant should insert curved forceps through the mouth and into the mid-cervical oesophagus.

2 The assistant should rotate the tip of the forceps laterally, until the point of the tips can be felt through the skin.

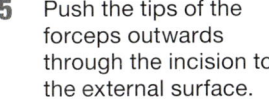

3 Make a 5–10 mm skin incision over this site.

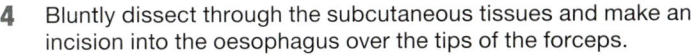

4 Bluntly dissect through the subcutaneous tissues and make an incision into the oesophagus over the tips of the forceps.

5 Push the tips of the forceps outwards through the incision to the external surface.

6 Measure the oesophagostomy tube from this point to the 9th rib (distal oesophagus). An assistant should mark this position on the tube with a permanent marker pen or piece of adhesive tape.

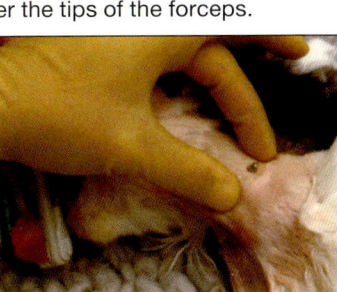

7 Open the tips of the forceps and grasp the distal end of the feeding tube.

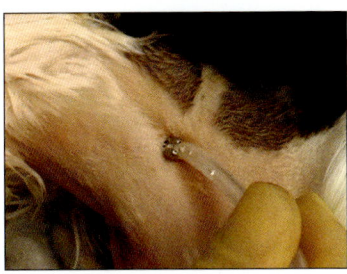

8 Draw the end of the tube through the oesophagostomy incision and rostrally into the pharynx to exit the mouth.

9 Disengage the tips of the forceps, and curl the tip of the tube back into the mouth.

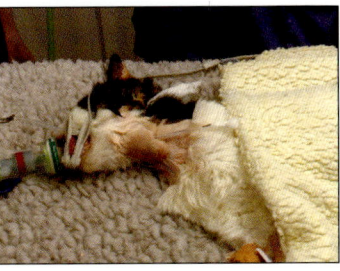

10 Feed the tube into the oesophagus while simultaneously pulling back the tube at the skin incision.

11 The tube should 'flip', causing it to pass caudally towards the stomach. Visually inspect the oropharynx, using a

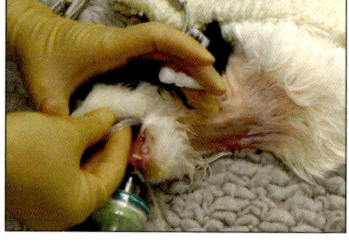

laryngoscope as required, to confirm that the tube is no longer present in the oropharynx.

12 The tube should slide easily back and forth a few centimetres, confirming that it has straightened.

13 Take a thoracic radiograph to confirm correct tube placement: the tip of the tube should be in the distal third of the oesophagus, not the stomach.

14 Secure the tube with a Chinese finger-trap suture.

15 Cover the tube site with a sterile dressing and place a soft, padded, loose, neck bandage.

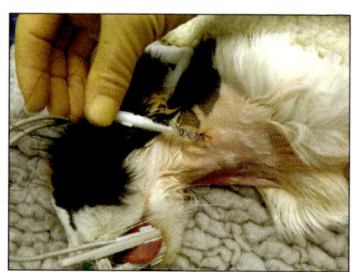

Using a percutaneous kit (van Noort technique)

1 An assistant should insert the rigid introducer through the mouth and into the mid-cervical oesophagus.

2 The assistant should rotate the introducer until the hole in its distal end can be felt through the skin.

3 Make a 5–10 mm skin incision over this site.

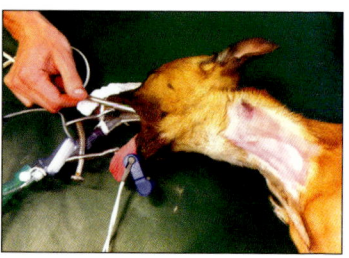

4 Introduce the needle and peel-away sheath as one unit through the skin incision, subcutaneous tissues and oesophageal wall, into the hole in the distal end of the rigid introducer.

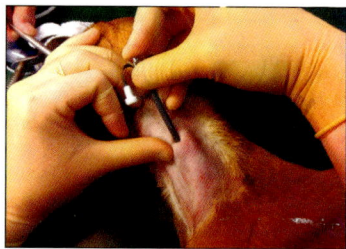

5 Whilst holding the sheath in place, remove the needle from the sheath.

6 Remove the rigid introducer.

7 Measure the oesophagostomy tube from the needle entry point to the 9th rib (distal oesophagus). An assistant should mark this position on the tube with a permanent marker pen or piece of adhesive tape.

8 Introduce the oesophagostomy tube through the sheath and into the oesophagus, stopping at the pre-marked length.

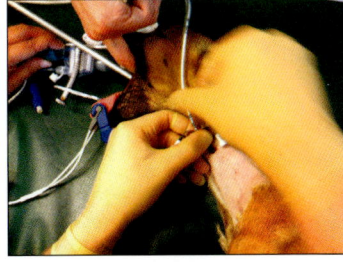

9 Grasping either side of the sheath, peel it away from the tube and remove it, to leave only the tube in place.

10 Take a thoracic radiograph to confirm correct tube placement: the tip of the tube should be in the distal third of the oesophagus, not the stomach.

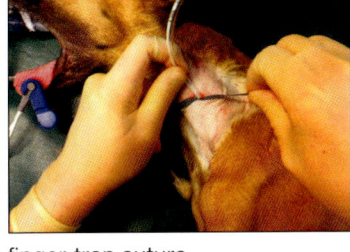

11 Secure the tube with a Chinese finger-trap suture.

12 Cover the tube site with a sterile dressing and place a soft, padded, loose, neck bandage.

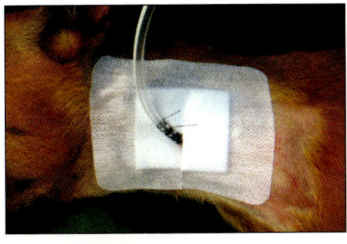
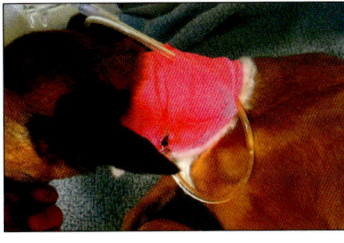

Feeding technique

> **NOTE**
>
> Feeding can commence as soon as the patient has recovered from general anaesthesia.

1 Instil sterile saline initially, in case the tube has migrated. If there is any doubt as to its position, take abdominal radiographs with or without sterile **iodinated contrast medium**.

2   Before feeding each time, flush the tube with small amounts (5–10 ml) of lukewarm tap water.

3   If the feeding tube is narrow bore, a liquid or semi-liquid food will be required.

4   Food should be warmed to body temperature and injected into the tube over approximately 5 minutes:

- Feed only one third of the resting energy requirement (RER) on the first day.
- On the second day, feed two-thirds of the RER, increasing to the entire RER on day three.
- Divide the daily requirement into multiple (5 or 6) feeds per 24 hours.

5   Flush the tube *after every feed* with 5–10 ml of lukewarm tap water.

RER

The resting energy requirement is now used as the 'baseline' energy recommendation for hospitalized dogs and cats, regardless of the disease or surgery.

The following equation can be used to calculate the RER in kcal/day for cats or dogs:

$$RER = 70 \times \text{bodyweight (kg)}^{0.75}$$

Alternatively, for animals >2 kg the following equation can be used:

$$RER = 30 \times \text{bodyweight (kg)} + 70$$

Note: To convert kcal to kilojoules (kJ) multiply by 4.185

Tube maintenance and removal

- Inspect and clean the stoma site daily, applying antibiotic cream if necessary. Apply a new sterile dressing and bandage.
- If the tube becomes blocked, 3 ml of a carbonated drink (e.g. cola or soda water) can be instilled and left for 5–10 minutes to help dislodge blockages.
- The tube can be removed when it is no longer required; there is no minimum length of time the tube must have been in place.
- To remove the tube, take off the bandage and sterile dressing, cut the suture and pull the tube out.
- The stoma site will close rapidly once the tube is removed. This should not be sutured.

Potential complications

- Major complications of feeding tube placement in dogs and cats are uncommon and can usually be avoided with proper technique and careful client counselling. The most common complications are:
  - Tube blockage
  - Infection at the tube site
  - Tube dislodgement or removal

Otoscopy

Indications/Use

- To obtain specimens for diagnosis of external ear canal disease
- To treat otitis externa. (For sampling and treating otitis media see **Myringotomy**)

Equipment

- Otoscope and cones of varying lengths and diameters OR a video-otoscope
- Cotton wool
- Haemostats for hair removal (if necessary)
- Sterile microbiology swab and transport medium
- Cotton wool buds
- Microscope slides
- 0.9% sterile saline
- 10 ml syringes
- Kidney dish
- Spruell needle or sterile catheters (e.g. 3.5 Fr tomcat catheter, long polypropylene catheter, 3.5 Fr feeding tube) of length sufficient to pass along the full length of the external ear canal

Patient preparation and positioning

- The animal can be examined standing, sitting or in lateral recumbency.
- Sedation or general anaesthesia may be required.
- Hair is removed, if necessary, by grasping groups of hairs with haemostats and twisting the handle.

Technique

1 Examine the pinnae and entrance to the ear canals with the naked eye.
2 Palpate the ear canal to evaluate pain, thickening and ossification of the ear canal. Note the presence of pus or cerumen. Examine each ear with the otoscope, starting with the normal ear if there is one. Apply lateral tension to the ear pinna with fingers to straighten the ear canal as the otoscope is advanced.
3 Visualize the tympanic membrane; in a normal ear this appears as a concave translucent membrane, with a dorsal, white, thick, well vascularized pars flaccida and a ventral semi-transparent pars tensa.
4 If significant pus or cerumen obscures evaluation of the ear canal or tympanic membrane, the ear can be flushed with lukewarm sterile saline. This is drawn into a 5–10 ml syringe attached to the Spruell needle or catheter, flushed into the ear canal, and re-aspirated. If possible, this is best performed under otoscopic visualization, with the needle or catheter passed through a side channel of the otoscope cone.

Sample handling

- Obtain samples for microbiological culture first. These can be collected using a sterile swab inserted through the sterile cone of an otoscope attachment, and then placed in transport medium for dispatch to the laboratory.
- To obtain cytology samples, a cotton bud or sterile swab is inserted down to the junction between the vertical and horizontal ear canals. The bud is rotated to collect debris:
  - This may be transferred to a slide with liquid paraffin and a coverslip applied prior to examination with a microscope, using low (4X objective) power
  - A smear can be made by rolling the cotton bud gently on to a microscope slide, and then air-dried and stained, as required.

Potential complications

- Rupture of tympanic membrane
- Injury to external ear canal

Pericardiocentesis

Indications/Use

- Relief of pericardial tamponade
- To obtain a sample of pericardial fluid for diagnostic evaluation

> **WARNING**
>
> - **Diuretics should NOT be given prior to pericardiocentesis. Not only will they be ineffective at relieving the clinical signs but the reduction in circulating fluid volume, and therefore intracardiac pressure, may exacerbate tamponade.**

Contraindications

- Suspected coagulopathy
- Active pericardial haemorrhage
- Severe arrhythmia

Equipment

- As required for **Aseptic preparation – (a) non-surgical procedures**
- A small-bore wire-guided drain, such as that used for **Thoracostomy tube placement – (b) small-bore wire-guided**
- OR a long (5–12.5 cm) wide-bore (14–18 G) over-the-needle catheter ± a narrow-gauge cat urinary catheter. *Note: check that the urinary catheter passes easily through the over-the-needle catheter before starting the procedure*
- OR a veterinary pericardial drainage catheter set (containing an 8.2 Fr, 20 cm long catheter with six distal side holes, an 18 G, 7 cm long introduction needle, and a 50 cm guidewire)
- Intravenous catheter, giving set and intravenous fluids
- Local anaesthetic
- No. 11 or 15 scalpel
- 3-way tap
- Extension tubing
- 20 ml syringe
- 50–60 ml syringe
- Measuring container
- EDTA and sterile plain collection tubes
- Microscope slides
- Suture materials or tissue glue
- ECG equipment

Patient preparation and positioning

- Sedation may be required to minimize movement.
- The animal is usually placed in sternal or left lateral recumbency, with **pericardiocentesis performed via a right-sided approach**. The procedure can be performed using a left-sided approach but is usually performed from the right side, to avoid the large coronary artery on the left and also to avoid the lungs by using the cardiac notch.

- Pericardiocentesis can be performed under ultrasound guidance, although the author's preference is to perform the procedure 'blind'.
- Place a peripheral **intravenous catheter** and give intravenous fluids to improve cardiac filling if required.
- The ECG leads are connected to the patient (see **Electrocardiography**).
- **Aseptic preparation – (a) non-surgical procedures** is performed on an area from the 3rd to the 7th rib, in the ventral half of the right chest wall.

Technique

1 The point of needle entry is approximately intercostal space 5 or 6, at the level of the costochondral junction. The exact site is located by palpating or auscultating where the cardiac impulse is strongest. Thoracic radiography or ultrasonography can also be used to indicate where the heart is most closely associated with the body wall and thus to determine the puncture site.

2 Infiltrate the skin and subcutaneous tissue with local anaesthetic.

3 Make a small stab incision through the skin with a scalpel blade.

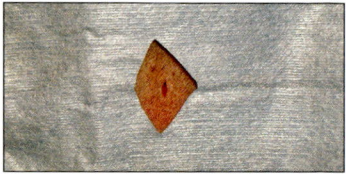

4 Three options are described: over-the-needle catheter (see below); wire-guided drain (see p. 197); and pericardial drainage set (see p. 198).

If using an over-the-needle catheter:

i   Insert the cannula and needle through the stab incision.

ii Slowly advance through the intercostal muscles just cranial to the rib (to avoid injury to the intercostal vessels) in a slightly cranial dorsal direction, until the tip of

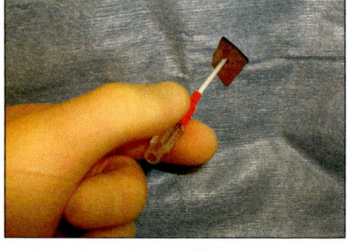

the needle reaches the visceral pericardium. With long-standing effusions there is often increased resistance and also a scratching sensation when the pericardial sac is first encountered.

iii A sharp stabbing motion may be required to penetrate the pericardium.

iv Pericardial fluid should appear in the hub. Pericardial fluid is typically quite haemorrhagic in dogs.

v   Advance the catheter over the needle and remove the needle.

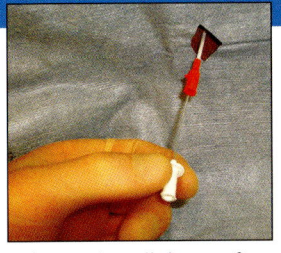
If using a small-bore wire-guided drain:

i   Insert the catheter introducer through the stab incision and advance as described above.

ii Once the introducer enters the pericardial sac and fluid is seen, advance the catheter completely into the pericardium over the needle and withdraw the needle.

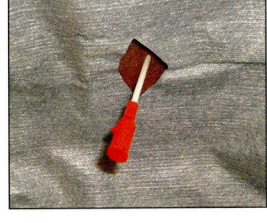

iii Thread the guidewire through the introducer catheter and into the pericardium.

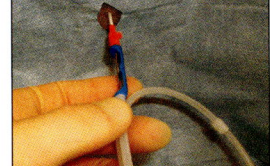

iv Advance the guidewire by approximately 10–20 cm. **The guidewire should be held at all times when it is partially within the pericardium.**

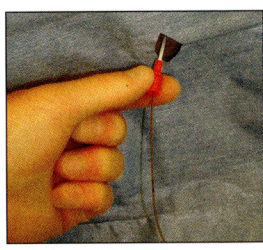

v   Remove the introducer catheter from the pericardium over the guidewire, leaving the guidewire in place within the pericardium.

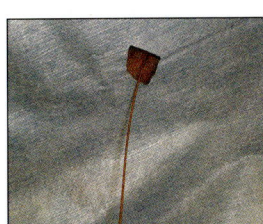

vi Advance the polyurethane catheter into the pericardium over the guidewire to the level of the suture wing.

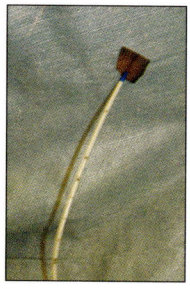

Introducing catheter.

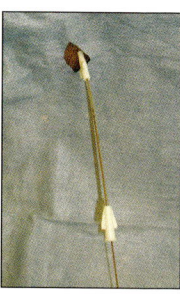

Catheter introduced.

vii Remove the guidewire.

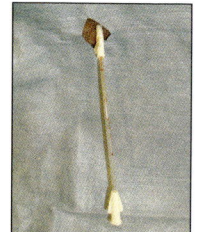

Guidewire removed.

If using a veterinary pericardial drainage catheter set:
Photos from BSAVA **companion** and courtesy of Luca Ferasin

i Attach a 20 ml syringe to the introduction needle.
ii Insert the introduction needle through the stab incision and advance the needle as described above, while maintaining a small vacuum in the 20 ml syringe.
iii Pericardial fluid should appear in the syringe.
iv Remove the syringe from the needle.
v Thread the guidewire (soft end) through the needle and into the pericardium. Advance the wire by approximately 10 cm. **The guidewire should be held at all times when it is partially within the pericardium.**

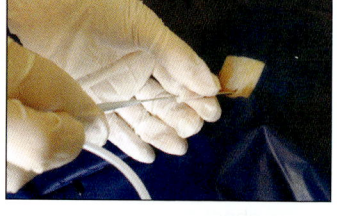

vi Remove the needle, leaving the guidewire in the pericardium.

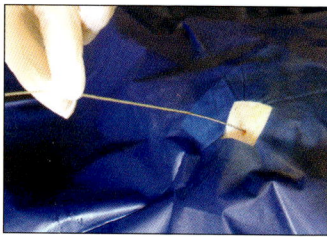

vii Thread the catheter over the guidewire, through the skin and intercostal space, and into the pericardium.

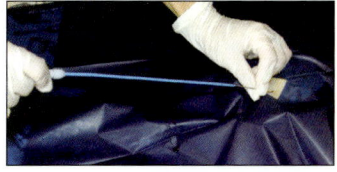

viii Remove the guidewire, leaving the catheter in the pericardium.

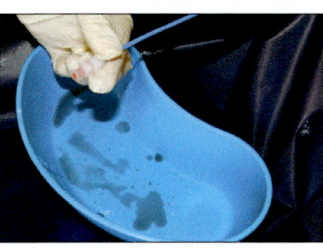

ARRHYTHMIAS

ECG monitoring throughout the procedure allows identification of arrhythmias caused by the catheter traumatizing the epicardium. Tachyarrhythmias (usually ventricular) are most commonly encountered. If these (or another arrhythmia) occur, the needle should be withdrawn slightly so that it no longer touches the epicardium.

5 Attach a 3-way tap, extension tubing and 50–60 ml syringe to create a closed drainage system, which can be operated by an assistant.

6 Aspirate the pericardial fluid.

7 If the flow of fluid stops, advance or withdraw the catheter by a few millimetres and re-aspirate, but avoid touching the epicardium.

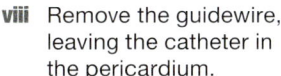

8 Place approximately 5 ml of pericardial fluid in a plain tube and observe for clot formation. If it clots, the fluid includes fresh blood and the procedure should be stopped. The PCV of the fluid (measured using a microcentrifuge) can also be checked to confirm that it is less than the PCV of peripheral blood.

9 Continue drainage until as much fluid as possible is removed. **NB** It is not necessary to drain the pericardial sac completely.

10 Place fluid into a measuring container and note the total volume.

11 After removal of the catheter, place a single suture in the skin incision if required, or close with tissue glue.

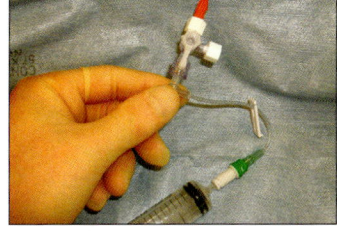

Sample handling

- Place the pericardial fluid in an EDTA tube for cytological analysis.
- Also make air-dried smears, especially if the sample is to be posted to an external laboratory.
- If there is a suspicion of infectious pericarditis, submit fluid in a sterile plain tube for bacteriological culture.

Potential complications

- Haemorrhage from the heart is uncommon and, if it occurs, is unlikely to result in catastrophic bleeding. The coronary arteries located on the right epicardium are relatively small, and the right ventricle is under relatively low pressure. Laceration of a cardiac tumour leading to haemorrhage can also occur
- It is common for arrhythmias to occur as the procedure is performed, but these do not usually cause clinically significant consequences
- Pneumothorax due to lung puncture

FURTHER INFORMATION

Management following pericardiocentesis is described in the *BSAVA Manual of Canine and Feline Emergency and Critical Care*. For interpretation of the results of fluid analysis see the *BSAVA Manual of Canine and Feline Clinical Pathology*.

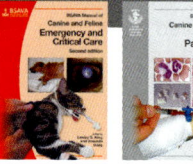

Peritoneal dialysis

Indications/Use

- Progressive azotaemia or severe intractable uraemia, primarily when this is due to acute kidney injury associated with oliguria (<0.25 ml/kg/h) or anuria
- Hyperkalaemia or other life-threatening electrolyte or acid–base disturbances
- Acute poisoning/drug overdose with substances that can be removed by dialysis, e.g. ethylene glycol, barbiturates, ammonia
- Life-threatening pulmonary oedema or iatrogenic fluid overload

---

PERITONEAL DIALYSIS OR HAEMODIALYSIS?

Peritoneal dialysis (PD) requires minimal specialized equipment and is not technically difficult. However, it is extremely labour-intensive, and close attention needs to be paid to the levels of sterility during the procedure. Haemodialysis is an alternative and superior technique and should be considered if available.

Contraindications

- Animals with chronic (end-stage) renal failure, as PD will only provide very short-term relief of clinical signs and/or a temporary reduction in the level of azotaemia
- Peritoneal fibrosis or adhesions that preclude solute exchange or prevent fluid distribution throughout the abdomen
- Severe coagulopathy
- Peritonitis
- Severe hypoalbuminaemia

Equipment

- As required for **Aseptic preparation – (b) surgical procedures**
- Commercial PD solution. *Alternatively*, a basic PD solution can be formulated by adding dextrose to lactated Ringer's solution (Hartmann's) (30ml of 50% dextrose in 1 litre = 1.5% dextrose solution). Dextrose can also be added at differing amounts to make approximate 2.5%, 3.5 or 4.25% solutions. The concentration of dextrose required depends on the hydration status of the patient; higher dextrose concentrations achieve improved ultrafiltration and water removal. A 4.25% solution should only be used when patients are fluid overloaded, and a 1.5% solution is generally adequate in normovolaemic patients. The addition of heparin (500 IU/l) to the dialysate is recommended for the first 24 hours following catheter placement to minimize the risk of catheter occlusion from fibrin deposition
- A PD catheter: The ideal catheter provides reliable, rapid dialysate flow rates without leaks or risk of infection. There are many catheter options, including commercial PD catheters such as the Tenckhoff catheter, the Blake silicone fluted drain, fluted-T catheters, the acute PD catheter, multipurpose tube catheters with stylet/trocar or Jackson–Pratt surgical suction drains.

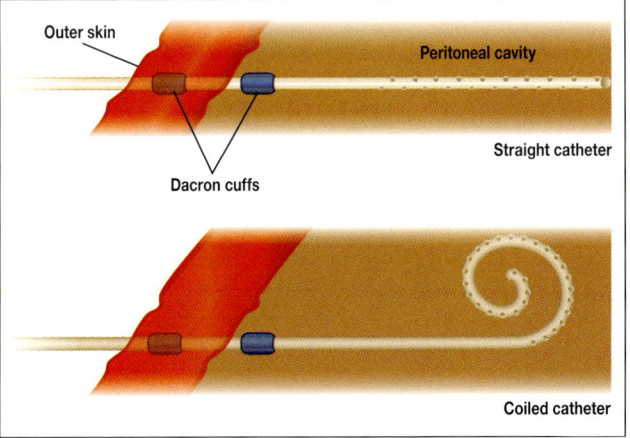

Tenckhoff catheter

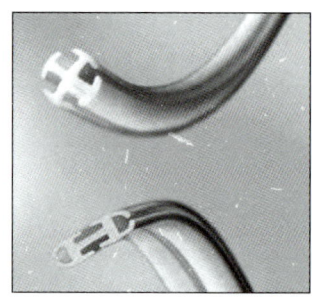

Blake silicone fluted drain

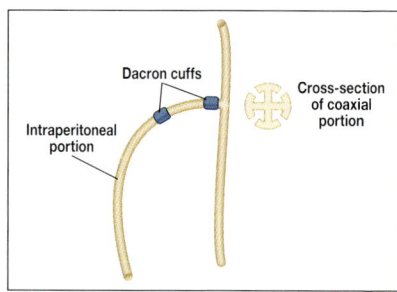

Fluted-T catheter

CATHETER/DRAIN OPTIONS

- Most commercial PD catheters are made of silicone rubber tubing or polyurethane, and have multiple fenestrations and one or more Dacron velour cuffs along the length of the tubing. The Dacron cuffs serve to anchor the catheter in place and provide a barrier to infection. Cuffs are positioned in the musculature ± the subcutaneous space, a few centimetres under the skin exit.
- A conventional straight Tenckhoff catheter is the most widely used catheter for PD in human patients.
- The optimal catheter type has not been established in veterinary medicine, although the fluted-T catheter has shown good results in dogs, and Blake silicon fluted drains have been used successfully for PD in cats.
- Fenestrated propylene peritoneal lavage catheters with an introduction needle and guidewire also exist for veterinary patients, although these are not designed to be left *in situ*.
- Jackson–Pratt surgical suction drains, placed by a mini-surgical approach, have been used in dogs and with less risk of occlusion than other multipurpose straight tube catheters. Several days of successful PD have been achieved using these drains and they are thus suitable alternatives if commercial PD catheters are not readily available.
- One of the authors [NB] has also used a 14 or 16 G chest tube, placed via Seldinger technique, for percutaneous peritoneal access for short-term (<24 hours) interim management, until a more 'permanent' catheter can be sourced; these catheters invariably kink and become obstructed within 12–24 hours.

- Urinary catheter (see **Urethral catheterization**)
- Local anaesthetic
- No. 11 or 15 scalpel
- Sterile surgical gloves

- Suture material
- Soft tissue surgical instrument set
- Commercial closed 'Y' system for drainage and infusion. *Alternatively,* a closed Y-system can be achieved using a 3-way tap, extension tubing and a collection bag such as an empty sterile fluid bag or urine collection bag
- 10–20 ml syringe
- Intravenous infusion pump

Patient preparation and positioning

- Depending on the temperament of the patient, light sedation may be required in order to minimize movement and avoid accidental bowel puncture.
- The patient is restrained in dorsal recumbency.
- **Aseptic preparation – (b) surgical procedures** is carried out over a large area of the abdomen from the xiphoid to the pubis, and a fenestrated drape placed.
- A **urinary catheter** should always be placed prior to PD catheter placement to prevent bladder trauma on PD catheter insertion.
- Administer a prophylactic dose of a first-generation cephalosporin prior to PD catheter insertion.

Technique

> **WARNING**
>
> - **Maintenance of sterility in connection, disconnection, infusion and drainage is of vital importance, since septic peritonitis is a relatively common and often lethal complication of PD. Sterile gloves should be worn during connection, disconnection and bag changes. Line connections should be covered with dressings soaked in povidone–iodine or chlorhexidine. Injection ports should be cleaned with chlorhexidine and alcohol prior to use.**

1 Infuse local anaesthetic into the skin, abdominal entry sites, and over the length of any planned subcutaneous tunnel. A subcutaneous tunnel should be made when placing any type of PD catheter, as this decreases the incidence of peritonitis and of dialysate leakage.

2 Techniques described for insertion of the PD catheter include: 'blind' percutaneous placement using a trocar or a guidewire (Seldinger technique); or a mini-surgical approach.

   If using a trocar: the site of catheter entry is on the midline or paramedian at the level of the umbilicus.
   i   Make a small skin incision (<0.4 cm) with a scalpel at this point.
   ii Advance the trocar and PD catheter into the abdomen by only 1–2 cm to avoid accidental laceration of abdominal organs.

iii   Once in the abdomen, the PD catheter is advanced off the stylet and directed caudally and positioned in the lower pelvis, in an unobstructed location.

iv   Once the intra-abdominal portion of the catheter has been placed, tunnel the distal tip of the catheter within the subcutaneous tissues.

If using a guidewire:

i   Make a small skin incision (<0.4 cm) with a scalpel at this point.

ii   Insert the catheter introducer into the abdomen and thread the guidewire through the introducer catheter in a caudal direction.

iii   Remove the introducer catheter from the guidewire, leaving the wire in place.

iv   Advance the PD catheter over the guidewire, again in a caudal direction, and position in the lower pelvis, in an unobstructed location.

v   Once the intra-abdominal portion of the catheter has been placed, tunnel the distal tip of the catheter within the subcutaneous tissues.

For a mini-surgical approach:

i   Abdominal penetration should be approximately 3–5 cm to the right of the midline, through the rectus muscle, at the level of the umbilicus. Make a 3–5 cm paramedian skin and subcutaneous incision.

ii   Make a 2–3 cm incision through the rectus muscle and into the abdominal cavity.

iii   A stay suture can be placed in the rectus sheath to allow manipulation of the body wall.

iv   Identify and incise the parietal peritoneum and direct the catheter caudally to position it in the lower pelvis, in an unobstructed location.

v   For snug abdominal wall closure, once the PD catheter exits the abdominal incision, the sterile distal end of the PD catheter is tunnelled immediately *under* the external sheath of the rectus abdominus muscle, through a segment of the muscle, prior to its exit through the subcutaneous tissues and skin.

vi   The rectus sheath is closed with a simple continuous or simple interrupted suture pattern using absorbable monofilament suture material.

vii   The skin is closed routinely over the abdominal insertion site.

3   Check catheter flow by connection to dialysate solution. A small volume of dialysate (10–20 ml) is infused into the abdomen in a sterile fashion. This small volume of dialysate should easily be retrieved to ensure unoccluded catheter placement; if not, the catheter should be redirected.

4 Secure the catheter at the skin exit site with a purse-string and finger trap suture.

5 Apply a non-occlusive sterile dressing, including several layers of sterile gauze, over the catheter exit site.

6 Once placed, attach the PD catheter to a commercial closed-Y connection system.

7 Infuse approximately 20 ml/kg of dialysate into the abdominal cavity by gravity flow or using an infusion pump over a 5–10 minute period.

8 Leave the dialysate in the abdomen for 30 minutes (the 'dwell' time). For dialysate retrieval, the collection system is placed below the patient and the fluid is allowed to drain by gravity over approximately 15 minutes. Drain as much fluid as possible.

> **NOTE**
>
> Throughout the dialysate infusion and dwell time, the patient must be monitored for any signs of discomfort, nausea or respiratory compromise, which would necessitate smaller infusion volumes.

9 Continue dialysate exchanges every 2 hours for the first 24–48 hours, or until the patient is clinically stable with blood urea nitrogen and creatinine levels in the lower half of the reference range.

10 Once patient improvement is noted, and target values are met, dialysis can be extended to every 4–6 hours. *For these later fluid exchanges, the dialysate should remain in the abdomen between exchanges (i.e. for 4–6 hours).*

11 PD should be continued until urine production is noted, renal function is adequate, and the patient is clinically improving. A specific creatinine value cannot be suggested, as animals will differ in their response to azotaemia.

> **PATIENT MONITORING**
>
> Careful monitoring of the patient and PD procedure is critical to delivery of effective and safe treatments, and allows complications to be addressed as early as possible. Critical monitoring data for patients are given in the table below. As a general rule of thumb, dialysate (effusate) volume should equal infused volume if a 1.25% dextrose solution is used, and effusate volume should be more than infused volume if a higher percentage dextrose solution is used for correction of overhydrated patients. Should effusate be less than infusate at any given cycle, consider patient hydration or catheter occlusion. Patient repositioning may also allow successful drainage. *continues ▶*

Physical examination parameters

- Bodyweight every 12 hours (same scales)
- Body temperature at least every 12 hours
- Exit site inspection every 24 hours
- Inspection for dialysate leakage or tunnel swelling/tenderness every exchange

Laboratory parameters

- Haematocrit and total protein every 12 hours
- Biochemistry panel every 24 hours
- Cytology of drained dialysate every 24 hours

Exchange parameters

- Drainage:
  - Start time
  - End time
  - Total drain time
  - Total drain volume
- Inflow:
  - Start time
  - End time
  - Total inflow time
  - Total volume infused
- Net balance per exchange (difference between outflow and prior inflow)

Potential complications

- Septic peritonitis
- Perforation of the intestines
- Subcutaneous dialysate leakage
- Wound infection
- Catheter occlusion
- Electrolyte disturbances
- Overhydration
- Protein loss/hypoalbuminaemia

Platelet count

Indications/Use

- Assessment of platelet numbers

Equipment

- Approximately 2 ml of *fresh* venous blood collected into an EDTA collection tube (see **Blood sampling – (b) venous**)
- Citrate collection tube

- Microhaematocrit tube
- Microscope slides
- 'Spreader' slide (as for **Blood smear preparation**)
- Stain (e.g. Diff-Quik)
- Microscope with oil immersion lens
- Immersion oil

Technique

1 Check the blood in the EDTA tube for clots. If clots are present, the subsequent count will be inaccurate; take a fresh sample.

> **NOTE**
>
> Blood can also be collected into citrate, as formation of platelet clumps may be reduced. However, collection into EDTA allows measurement of other haematological variables.

2 Make a **blood smear** and stain with a suitable stain.

3 Examine the feathered edge of the blood smear for platelet clumps.

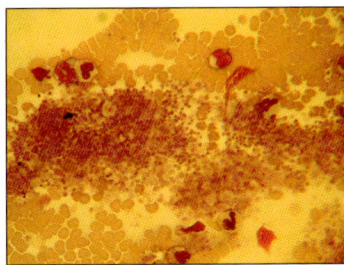

If clumps are present, the subsequent count will be inaccurate; take a fresh sample and repeat 1–3.

4 Identify an area of the smear, away from the feathered edge, where there is a monolayer of evenly distributed cells.

5 Count the platelets in 5 high-power fields (1000X, oil-immersion) and calculate the average.

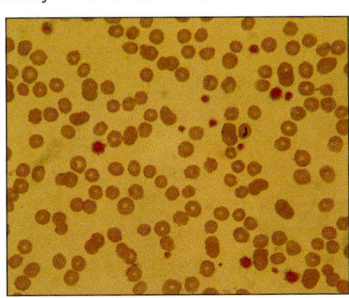

There are 14 platelets in this hpf.

Reference ranges

- Approximately 1 platelet per high-power field is equivalent to 15×10^9 platelets per litre in dogs and cats.
- The normal reference range for platelets in dogs and cats is $>200 \times 10^9/l$.

Prostatic wash

Indications/Use

To obtain a sample for cytology and bacteriological culture from dogs with:

- Prostatomegaly
- Other abnormalities in shape, symmetry or consistency of the prostate
- Prostatic pain
- Haematuria or pyuria

Equipment

- Sterile male dog urinary catheter
- 4% chlorhexidine gluconate
- Bowl to collect urine
- Sterile 0.9% saline
- 2 and 5 ml syringes
- EDTA and sterile plain collection tubes
- Microscope slides

Patient preparation and positioning

- Can be performed on the conscious dog, although light sedation is generally preferable.
- The patient is placed in lateral recumbency.
- The prepuce must be cleaned of all debris, using dilute chlorhexidine, and rinsed with warm water.

Technique

1   Using an aseptic technique, introduce a urinary catheter and empty the bladder of urine (see **Urethral catheterization**).
2   The bladder should also be flushed with saline and emptied again to ensure that all urine has been removed. A sample of the saline flush can be collected and handled as below, for comparison with the prostatic wash to help clarify the site of pathology (bladder *versus* prostate).
3   Perform a rectal examination, or alternatively an assistant can perform the rectal examination.
4   Partially withdraw the catheter to the level of the prostate, guiding the catheter per rectum.
5   Massage the prostate per rectum or transabdominally (if the prostate cannot be palpated per rectum) for 1 minute and at the same time slowly inject 1–2 ml of sterile saline into the urinary catheter.
6   After a further minute's massage, using a 5 ml syringe aspirate material into the catheter and syringe. The catheter can also be passed into the bladder and the prostatic wash fluid aspirated from there.
7   Remove the syringe from the catheter when sufficient material has been collected.

8   Repeat steps 5 and 6 if an insufficient sample has been collected.
9   Remove the catheter.
10 Fill the syringe with air and expel any remaining fluid from the catheter into the collection tubes or on to a microscope slide.

Sample handling

- Place an aliquot in an EDTA tube for cytology.
- Submit a portion of the sample in a sterile plain tube for culture if infection is suspected.
- If samples are to be sent to an external laboratory, fresh air-dried unstained smears of any flocculent/mucoid material should also be made (see **Fine needle aspiration**). Direct smears of the fluid can also be made, but most samples are poorly cellular.

Potential complications

- Rupture of prostatic abscess
- Rectal perforation
- Ascending urinary tract infection

Retrograde urethrography/ vaginourethrography

Indications/Use

- Haematuria
- Dysuria
- Stranguria
- Urinary incontinence
- Urethral discharge
- Urethral trauma

Equipment

- Water-soluble, **iodinated contrast medium** (150–200 mg iodine/ ml; more concentrated solutions can be diluted with normal saline). This contrast can be mixed with an equal volume of sterile jelly (e.g. K-Y) to produce a more viscous medium and better urethral distension. This mixture should be made up well in advance, since small air bubbles introduced at mixing can mimic genuine filling defects due to calculi. It should be stored in a dark place as iodinated media degrade in light
- Local anaesthetic
- Wide-bore male dog urinary catheters of appropriate size for male dogs, or tomcat catheters of appropriate size for male cats. Catheters should fit snugly to limit leakage of contrast out of the urethra (see **Urethral catheterization**)
- Foley urinary catheters of appropriate size for bitches and queens (see **Urethral catheterization**)
- Tongue forceps or bowel clamps

Patient preparation and positioning

- Urethrography is best performed under general anaesthesia, especially in females.
- The patient is positioned for **Urethral catheterization**.

Technique

Retrograde urethrography (males)

1 The urethral area should be assessed on plain radiographs for evidence of soft tissue swelling or the presence of radiopaque calculi *prior* to performing contrast studies. A pneumocystogram can be performed, to produce back pressure against which to distend the urethra, but this is not advised in cases of suspected urethral or bladder rupture.

2 Catheterize the urethra with the widest catheter possible, prefilled with saline to avoid producing air bubbles.

3 Position the tip of the catheter distal to the area under investigation.

4 In **cats**, the catheter does not need to be secured in position. In **dogs**, hold the penis tightly around the catheter: this can be performed with tongue forceps. Local anaesthetic can be

instilled into the urethral catheter prior to contrast medium, to reduce muscle spasm.

5   Inject up to 1 ml/kg of the diluted contrast medium as a bolus, avoiding excessive pressure.

6   Take radiographs immediately after injecting. Lateral views are usually most helpful. Ventrodorsal views can give extra information about the prostatic urethra: slight obliquity from the ventrodorsal position will avoid superimposition of the urethra over itself or over bony structures.

Retrograde vaginourethrography (females)

1   The urethral area should be assessed on plain radiographs for evidence of soft tissue swelling or the presence of radiopaque calculi *prior* to performing contrast studies. A pneumocystogram can be performed, to produce back pressure against which to distend the urethra, but this is not advised in cases of suspected urethral or bladder rupture.

2   Cut the tip off the Foley catheter, beyond the inflatable bulb, to prevent it passing too far into the vagina; in cats, a non-cuffed catheter is often used.

3   Prefill the catheter with saline and place the catheter tip just inside the vulval lips, holding the vulva closed around the catheter using, for example, gentle bowel clamps or tongue forceps.

4   Inflate the bulb of the catheter.

5   Inject a little local anaesthetic and then the diluted water-soluble contrast medium. Dose rate is up to 1 ml/kg over 5–10 seconds. Take care to avoid vaginal rupture.

6   Take radiographs immediately after injecting. Lateral views are standard but an oblique ventrodorsal view (to avoid superimposition of the vagina and urethra) may also be helpful.

Potential complications

- Urinary tract infection
- Urethral rupture

Rhinoscopy

Indications/Use

- Investigating clinical signs of nasal disease
- Investigating dysphagia, head shaking, exophthalmos, facial swelling or deformity, pawing at the nose and halitosis in the absence of dental disease
- Foreign body removal
- Collecting samples for histology, cytology and microbiology

Contraindications

- Inadequate investigations prior to endoscopy
- Coagulopathy
- Severe hypertension

Equipment

- Caudal rhinoscopy: *flexible* endoscope (diameter 3.5–6 mm)
- Anterior rhinoscopy: *flexible* (as above) *or rigid* endoscope (diameter 2.4–2.7 mm, 0–30 degrees) with sheath or cannula to allow fluid irrigation
- Endoscopic viewing equipment
- 1 litre bags of 0.9% saline (pre-warmed to 37°C) and fluid giving set for irrigation
- Pharynx packs. These can be made by rolling up pieces of gauze swab and tying a gauze bandage around the roll; the swab can be packed in the caudal pharynx, whilst the bandage should remain outside the mouth to allow easy retrieval. Alternatively, a small sponge with a tie attached can be used

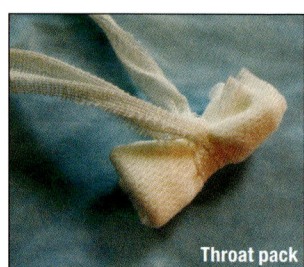

Throat pack

- Mouth gag
- Local anaesthetic spray
- Water-soluble lubricant (e.g. K-Y jelly)
- 7 Fr 20–40 cm grasping forceps
- Spay hook
- Flexible cup-style biopsy forceps that can pass through the biopsy channel of the rigid endoscope, or 3–5 mm rigid biopsy forceps
- 10–20 ml syringes
- Sterile kidney dish
- Container with 10% neutral buffered formalin
- Hypodermic needle: 21 or 23 G
- Tissue cassette with foam insert ('cell-safe' frames)
- EDTA, sterile plain tubes and microscope slides

Patient preparation and positioning

- **General anaesthesia is essential**. Always place a *cuffed* endotracheal (ET) tube.
- The patient should be placed in sternal recumbency, with the head propped up slightly to elevate the mouth and nasal planum for ease of access. The nose can be angled downwards to direct liquid away from the pharynx.
- There is a strong gag reflex present when performing caudal rhinoscopy. This is normal and does not necessarily mean that the animal is not anaesthetized deeply enough. The use of topical local anaesthetic spray on the mucosal surfaces may help to blunt this reflex.
- A mouth gag is essential when performing *caudal* rhinoscopy, to keep the mouth open and prevent the patient biting the endoscope in the event that contact with the pharynx stimulates a gag reflex.
- The procedure is best performed on a 'wet table', due to the large volume of irrigant used. Towels placed on the floor are useful to catch additional spillage.

> **WARNING**
>
> ■ Care should be exercised if using cold irrigant solutions, especially in small patients. The high surface area and excellent vascular supply of the nares act like a heat sink, and can result in hypothermia. Careful monitoring of body temperature is advisable.

Technique

> **NOTE**
>
> It is good practice to examine the nasopharynx and choanae using caudal (posterior) rhinoscopy *before* performing the rostral (anterior) procedure. Caudal rhinoscopy is performed by retroflexing a flexible endoscope over the free edge of the soft palate, so as to look forward, towards the choanae. Since this does not require fluid irrigation, samples can be obtained for culture if required, as well as biopsy samples of nasopharyngeal and caudal nasal masses.

Caudal (posterior, retropharyngeal) rhinoscopy

1 Insert the flexible endoscope into the mouth.

2 Advance the endoscope caudally and pass the free edge of the soft palate.

3 Retroflex the endoscope into a 'J' position behind the soft palate to view the nasopharynx.

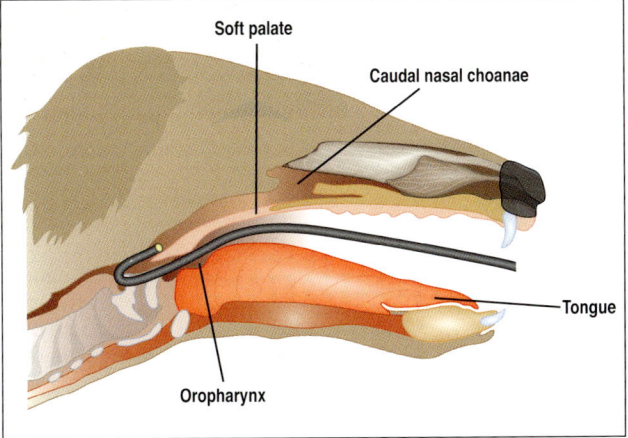

4 Gradually withdraw the endoscope rostrally, with the tip still flexed, to advance the tip toward the choanae.

5 As the endoscope is retroflexed, the view on the monitor is upside down and reversed: up is down; and left is right.

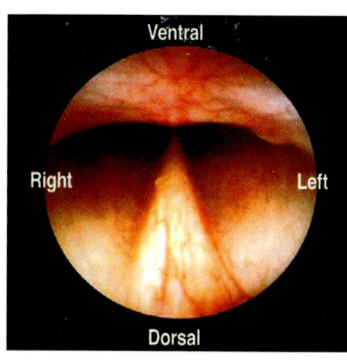

Ventral

Right   Left

Dorsal

(Courtesy of
RC Denovo)

Anterior (rostral) rhinoscopy

1 Place a swab pack in the caudal pharynx and ensure the cuff of the ET tube is inflated. Alternatively, a bandage roll can be used. Large volumes of fluid will be washed over the soft palate and there will be a continuous flow of saline through the nose and out of the mouth. Swabs should be counted and recorded.

2 Begin with the normal or less affected side.

3 Coat the shaft of the endoscope sheath/cannula with water-soluble lubricant, being careful not to get any on the lens of the endoscope.

4 Hold the endoscope in a 'pistol' fashion, with the light guide cable and port facing the floor, and the camera oriented such that any graphics on the camera head can be read right side up. This will ensure that the image produced on the monitor is true.

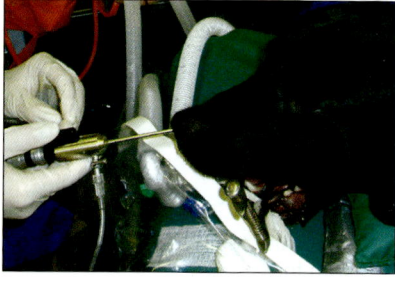

5 Deflect the nasal planum dorsally and introduce the rigid endoscope with its sheath ventromedially (toward the base of the opposite ear) so that it will pass into the ventral meatus of the nasal cavity.

6 With a bag of saline and giving set connected to one of the stopcocks of the cannula, start the flow of fluid. This is often needed to remove the copious discharge or haemorrhage that obscures the view. Control of saline is best adjusted with the tap on the ingress port of the rhinoscope, so the controls on the giving set may be left open.

7 Whilst pointing the endoscope ventrally and medially, advance the endoscope caudally while examining the turbinates of the ventral meatus.

8 Pass the endoscope to the level of the posterior nares and nasopharynx.

9 On entering the nasopharynx, just caudal to the posterior nares, the orifice of the eustachian tube can be seen on the lateral wall.

10 Retract the endoscope rostrally and examine the dorsal meatus
and ethmoid turbinates.

11 Ensure that all swabs or the bandage roll are removed from the
pharynx before recovery of the patient from anaesthesia.

Biopsy and sampling

- Samples should *always* be taken, even if no lesions are apparent.
  In addition to biopsy samples, brushings and swabs may also be
  taken for cytology or culture.

- It is important to perform *biopsy at multiple sites*, as there is little
  correlation between visual appearance and specific disease
  entities.

- The operator can use:
  - Flexible cup-style biopsy forceps introduced via the biopsy
    channel of the endoscope
  - Rigid biopsy forceps passed alongside the shaft of the
    endoscope
  - Nasal flush (for cytology).

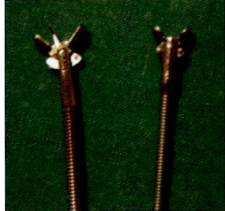

Flexible cup-style

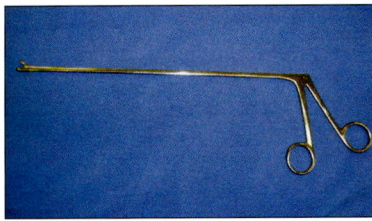

Rigid

Using flexible cup-style biopsy forceps

1 Position the tip of the endoscope approximately 3–5 cm rostral
to the lesion to be sampled.

2 Insert the forceps through the biopsy channel of the endoscope,
with the cup firmly closed, and advance them towards the site of
interest. Note that forceps should not be passed down the
biopsy channel of a flexible endoscope when it is in a 'J' position.
Instead, the flexible endoscope should be straightened, the
forceps passed down the biopsy channel until they protrude a
short distance from the end, and the endoscope then returned to
the 'J' position.

3 Once the forceps have passed out of the end of the endoscope,
open the cup, advance on to the region to be sampled, and close
the cups.

4 Withdraw the forceps from the endoscope and gently remove
the sample.

Using rigid biopsy forceps

1 Position the tip of the endoscope approximately 3–5 cm rostral
to the lesion to be sampled.

2 Pass the forceps along the dorsal edge of the rhinoscope,
opposite the light guide post, to the site of interest.

■ The tips of the rigid biopsy forceps must not pass beyond the level of the medial canthus of the eyes. Measure the distance between the tip of the rhinarium and the medial canthus, and mark it with a piece of sticky tape on the forceps themselves to prevent inadvertent penetration of the cribriform plate.

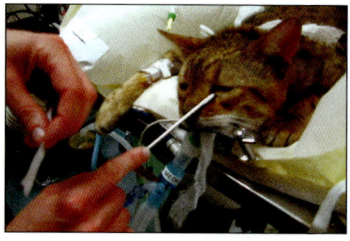

■ In smaller patients, where it is not possible to pass the forceps alongside the endoscope, it is useful to measure the position of the lesion by assessing the direction and depth of the tip of the endoscope, and taking samples 'blind'.

3 Once the tips have passed the end of the endoscope, open the tips, advance on to the region to be sampled, and close the tips.

4 Withdraw the forceps and gently remove the sample.

Nasal flush

1 Pack the caudal pharynx with swabs or a bandage roll.

2 Fill several 20 ml syringes with saline (10 ml syringes for a cat or a dog <5 kg).

3 Wedge the nozzle of the syringe into one nostril and occlude the contralateral nostril.

4 Holding an empty sterile kidney dish below the nostrils, empty the syringe with moderate force into one nostril.

5 Repeat several times for both nostrils. Usually, foreign bodies and many mass lesions will be dislodged with two or three attempts.

6 Ensure that all swabs or the bandage roll are removed from the pharynx before recovery of the patient from anaesthesia. Examine these for any foreign material or dislodged tissue.

Sample handling

■ To remove samples from the biopsy forceps, immerse in 10% neutral buffered formalin. Then rinse the forceps in saline before reinserting them into the endoscope.

■ *Alternatively,* carefully remove samples from the biopsy forceps with a needle and place directly into 10% neutral buffered formalin, or lay on the foam insert of a tissue cassette.

■ Place tissue samples for bacterial or fungal culture on a bacterial transport swab or in a sterile container.

■ Portions of tissue samples can be used to make impression smears for cytological assessment.

■ Place nasal flush samples into an EDTA tube for cytology, and into a sterile plain tube for bacterial culture, if required.

■ To minimize cellular degradation, it is preferable to make direct smears of any mucoid material retrieved from a nasal flush and send these to the laboratory unstained.

Foreign body removal

- Cats: Tend to be presented with nasopharyngeal foreign bodies that have been coughed up and lodged over the free edge of the soft palate. These can often be removed without the use of an endoscope, using rigid grasping forceps. A spay hook to retract the soft palate rostrally can also aid removal.
- Dogs: More prone to foreign bodies in the nasal cavities. If small, these can be removed under endoscopic guidance using rigid grasping forceps. Larger foreign bodies will require 'blind' removal with rigid grasping forceps.
- If the foreign body breaks up and is impossible to remove completely, the nose should be flushed vigorously with sterile saline. The throat pack should be pushed caudally beyond the tip of the soft palate to allow this fluid to drain over the soft palate and into the mouth freely; lower the nose to allow drainage.

Potential complications

- Significant mucosal haemorrhage is rare; if it does occur, pressure can be placed over the rostral nares whilst occluding the caudal pharynx with swabs. *Alternatively,* adrenaline can be sprayed into the nares using a urinary catheter or over-the-needle catheter and syringe
- Penetration of the cribriform plate is uncommon unless significant disease is present, and/or the biopsy forceps are passed 'blind' or beyond the level of the medial canthus of the eyes

Seizures – emergency protocol

> **NOTE**
>
> ■ An *integrated approach* to patients in status epilepticus can achieve emergency stabilization, therapeutic intervention and diagnostic investigation *simultaneously*.
> ■ Although immediate anticonvulsant therapy and systemic stabilization are warranted, concurrent history taking, physical examination and diagnostic tests may be useful.

Systemic stabilization

- **A**   Airway: intubate if necessary.
- **B**   Breathing: administer 100% oxygen via a non-rebreathing mask.
- **C**   Circulation: place a large **intravenous catheter**; *once seizures have stopped*, start on isotonic saline (10 ml/kg/h).
- Temperature regulation: treat hyperthermia promptly with slow passive cooling if >40°C; stop at 38.5°C to prevent hypothermia.

Drug therapy

1   Diazepam: 0.5–1.0 mg/kg i.v. or per rectum
    OR
    Midazolam: 0.2–0.3 mg/kg i.v. or i.m.
2   If seizures persist: repeat step 1 up to three times every 3 minutes
    AND
    Begin loading with phenobarbital (also known as phenobarbitone). Monitor respiration, blood pressure and oxygen saturation, as phenobarbital can suppress cardiorespiratory function.
    - Phenobarbital-naïve patient:
        - Phenobarbital loading dose: 24 mg/kg i.v. over 24 hours.
        - Divide into doses of 3–5 mg/kg i.v. and give every 30 min to every 4 h to effect
          OR
          Give 4 mg/kg/h i.v. continuous rate infusion, but total dose rate must not exceed 100 mg/min
    - Patient that is currently receiving phenobarbital treatment:
        - 2–4 mg/kg i.v. or i.m. as a single bolus.
3   If seizures persist, **one or more** of the following treatments may be used:
    - Propofol: 6 mg/kg i.v. given as 1–2 mg/kg boluses to effect, followed by 0.1–0.2 mg/kg/min i.v. continuous rate infusion

- Diazepam: 0.5 mg/kg/h i.v. continuous rate infusion. Dilute diazepam in 5% dextrose or 0.9% saline.
- Levetiracetam: 40–60 mg/kg i.v. or per rectum, followed by 20 mg/kg i.v. every 8 hours
- Ketamine (last resort): 5 mg/kg i.v. bolus, followed by 5 mg/kg/h i.v. continuous rate infusion.

Diagnostics

- Glucose analysis: if hypoglycaemic, treat with 50% dextrose diluted to 25% (500 mg/kg i.v.) over 15 minutes or treat with oral glucose syrup; if hyperglycaemic, monitor effects of fluid therapy once the seizures have stopped.
- Electrolyte analysis: treat immediately with fluid therapy.
- Arterial blood gas: marked metabolic acidosis is common and will resolve following stabilization; however, respiratory acidosis needs immediate treatment.
- Haematology/serum chemistry: can be affected by seizure activity, so may need to repeat 48 hours after stabilization.
- Urinalysis: rule out myoglobinuria and monitor urine output with indwelling catheter.
- ECG: arrhythmias can occur up to 72 hours after the seizures due to myocardial damage.
- Whole blood ammonia concentrations and/or bile acid stimulation test: to check for hepatic encephalopathy.
- Toxicity screen: immediate results will not be available but take blood to submit for cholinesterase levels after stabilization.
- **Cerebrospinal fluid sampling**: rule out inflammatory disease.
- MRI/CT scan: rule out structural disease.
- Anti-epileptic drug blood levels.

History

- When did the episode start?
- Is there a pre-existing seizure disorder?
- Is the patient on anticonvulsant therapy? If so, what is the dose; when was the last dose; have serum anticonvulsant levels been measured recently?
- Is the patient on any other medications?
- Are there any systemic health problems?
- Has there been a recent change in personality or behaviour?
- Has there been any recent trauma, travel history or toxin exposure?
- Has the patient eaten a meal within the last few hours?

Physical examination

- Complete physical examination.

Skin biopsy – punch biopsy

Indications/Use

- Obtaining a full-thickness skin sample in cases of diffuse dermatosis, in particular:
    - Suspected dermatosis with a characteristic histopathology, e.g. follicular dysplasia, sebaceous adenitis, dermatomyositis, immune-mediated disease
    - Dermatoses that fail to respond to appropriate rational therapy
    - Any dermatosis that appears unusual or particularly severe
- Punch biopsy is less useful for ulcers and nodules, as it is difficult to straddle the margin or encompass the lesion

Contraindications

- Coagulopathy
- History of poor wound healing
- Punch biopsy is inappropriate for masses or the junctional area between affected and non-affected skin: an excisional biopsy would be preferred in these instances

Equipment

- 6–8 mm biopsy punch (a 4 mm punch can be used for restricted sites, such as nose and paws)
- Curved scissors for hair
- 70% surgical spirit
- Local anaesthetic: 2% lidocaine
- Fine forceps
- Mayo scissors
- No. 11 scalpel
- Containers containing 10% neutral buffered formalin
- Sterile containers for specimens for culture
- Sterile 0.9% saline
- Pieces of card approximately 10 x 10 mm
- Suture material (monofilament nylon), needle and needle holders for skin closure

Patient preparation and positioning

- Punch biopsy can usually be performed under light sedation, using local anaesthesia.
- General anaesthesia is required for sensitive sites, such as the face and feet, where local anaesthesia is difficult.
- The patient should be positioned with the area to be sampled uppermost.
- Any hair at the biopsy site should be cut with curved scissors, without disturbing the skin surface.
- Minimal skin preparation is required, though the skin should first be wiped with 70% surgical spirit if the sample is to be sent for culture.

Technique

1 Infiltrate the skin and subcutis with 0.5–1 ml of 2% lidocaine.
2 Press the biopsy punch firmly against the skin and rotate in one direction.
3 Using fine forceps, lift the base clear and cut it free, using Mayo scissors or a scalpel blade.

> **WARNING**
> - **Do not grasp the skin sample itself, as this will cause crush artefacts.**

4 Close the skin defect; a single interrupted suture is usually sufficient.

Sample handling

- Place the biopsy specimen, subcutis down, on a piece of card. On the other end of the card, draw a circle with an arrow through it to indicate the direction of hair growth.
- Place the biopsy specimen in a container of 10% neutral buffered formalin.
- Specimens for bacterial or fungal culture should be submitted in a sterile container with 2–3 drops of sterile saline to prevent drying in transit.
- Submit each biopsy specimen in a separate, clearly labelled pot to avoid any confusion.

Potential complications

- Bleeding should cease with pressure; continued haemorrhage may suggest a coagulopathy
- Delayed wound healing

Soft padded bandage

Indications

- To control limb oedema and swelling
- To support the limb following surgery

Equipment

- Adhesive tape (2.5 cm wide)
- Tongue depressor (optional)
- Cast padding or cotton roll
- Conforming gauze bandage
- Outer protective bandage material (e.g. self-adhesive, non-adherent bandage)

Patient preparation and positioning

- Sedation or general anaesthesia may be required where the limb is painful or the animal is non-compliant.
- The animal should be placed in lateral recumbency with the affected limb uppermost.
- The affected limb should be supported in a weight-bearing position, and an appropriate dressing placed directly over any wounds or surgical incisions.

Technique

1 Place two strips of adhesive tape (stirrups) on the distal limb, on *either* the dorsal and palmar/plantar surfaces *or* the medial and lateral surfaces. These tape strips extend beyond the tip of the toes and are stuck to each other or to a tongue depressor.

2 Beginning distally, apply cast padding material or cotton roll up the limb, in a spiral fashion, overlapping the layers by 50%. The bottom of the bandage should be at the level of the nailbeds of digits III and IV.

3 Place conforming gauze snugly over the cotton layer, again overlapping layers by 50%. The conforming gauze should compress the cotton but not create venous stasis. It should not extend proximally beyond the level of the cotton.

4 Separate the tape stirrups, rotate them through 180 degrees, and apply them proximally to the bandage to limit slippage. The pads and nails of the axial digits should remain exposed.

5 Apply an outer protective bandage material to the bandage. This should not be applied tightly: it should be pulled free from the roll, the tension released from the material, and the material simply placed over the gauze.

Robert Jones technique

- The Robert Jones bandage is a heavily padded modification, which provides effective support for the first aid management of distal limb fractures.
- It is only suitable for fractures distal to the elbow in the forelimb and distal to the stifle in the hindlimb.
- For fractures of the humerus or femur, the distal edge of the Robert Jones bandage acts as a fulcrum, across which the fracture pivots, with the possibility of exacerbating soft tissue injury and further fracture displacement.
- One version of the Robert Jones bandage can be achieved by applying three consecutive layers of cast padding material or cotton roll, each of which is compressed with a layer of conforming gauze. The Robert Jones bandage is protected by a final layer of an outer protective bandage material. Bandage materials are applied to the limb as for the soft padded bandage.

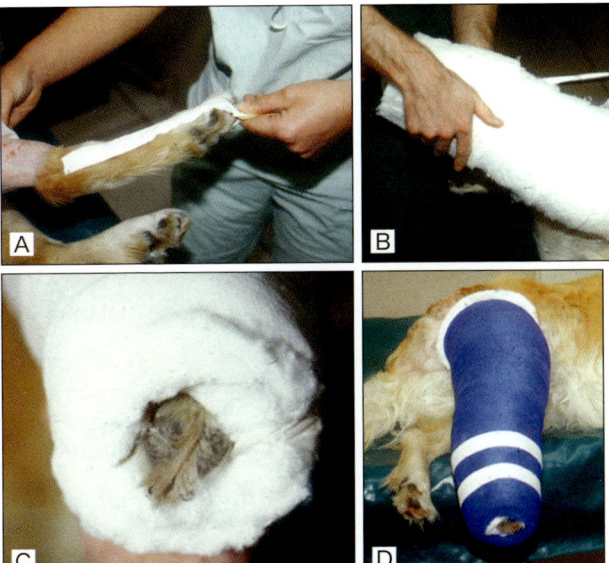

Robert Jones bandage. **A** Applying traction tapes. **B** Cotton wool around the limb.
C Exposed toes. **D** Cohesive bandage in place.

Bandage care and maintenance

- Soft padded bandages should be checked every 4 hours for the first 24 hours and at least twice daily thereafter for complications.
- Written instructions should always be given to clients at discharge; owners must understand their responsibility regarding bandage maintenance.
- Exercise restriction is generally indicated.
- The bandaged limb should be monitored for swollen toes, cold toes, wetness, soiling or slippage, and changed if necessary.
- The bandage must be kept clean and dry. A plastic bag may be placed over the foot while the animal is walking outside and then removed when it is indoors.
- If no open wounds are present, the bandage may be changed every 7–10 days. If open wounds are present, the bandage should be changed as needed, sometimes several times daily.
- In young, rapidly growing animals the bandage should be changed every 4–5 days.

Potential complications

- Venous stasis
- Limb oedema
- Moist dermatitis
- Maceration of skin underlying a wet bandage
- Contamination of wounds
- Pressure necrosis
- Skin irritation at the site of the tape stirrups

Spica splint

Indications/Use

- Support of the elbow following:
    - Closed reduction of traumatic **elbow luxation** with or without open repair of collateral ligament injuries
    - Internal fixation of olecranon fractures
- Support of the shoulder following closed reduction of traumatic lateral shoulder luxation

Equipment

- Adhesive tape (2.5 cm wide)
- Cast padding
- Conforming gauze bandage
- Resin-impregnated fibreglass cast materials
- Outer protective bandage material (e.g. self-adhesive non-adherent bandage or adhesive bandage)

Patient preparation and positioning

- The animal should be sedated heavily or under general anaesthesia.
- The animal should be placed in lateral recumbency, with the affected limb uppermost and supported in a weight-bearing position.
- For large breed dogs, lying the dog across two tables, such that the thorax is accessible between them, facilitates the placement of this dressing without the need to lift the dog multiple times.

Technique

1   Apply a light Robert Jones **soft padded bandage**, *excluding* the final outer bandage layer, to the entire forelimb and extend this bandage over the dorsal midline to encompass the thorax. Take care not to apply the bandage too tightly to the thorax, so as not to compromise respiration.

2   Follow the manufacturer's recommendations regarding wetting and handling of the cast material.

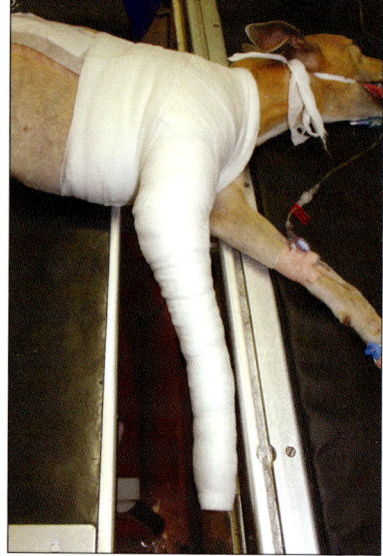

3 Apply strips of cast material over the lateral aspect of the bandage. These strips should extend from the distal tip of the bandage to proximally over the dorsal midline to the contralateral scapula. Cast material should be conformed to the contours of the limb and thorax.

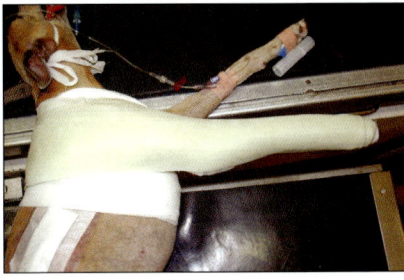

4 Secure the cast material to the underlying Robert Jones bandage with an outer protective bandage material.

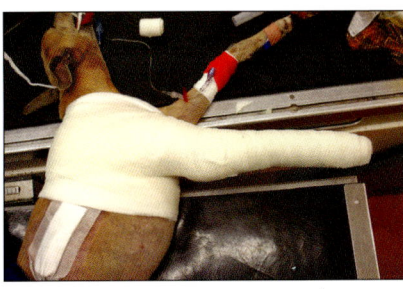

Splint care and maintenance

- Written instructions should always be given to clients at discharge; owners must understand their responsibility in splint maintenance.
- Exercise restriction must be enforced.
- Spica splints should be checked every 4 hours for the first 24 hours and then at least twice daily thereafter for complications.
- The limb should be monitored for swollen toes, cold toes or skin abrasions. The splint should be monitored for wetness, soiling or slippage, and changed if necessary.
- The splint must be kept clean and dry. A plastic bag may be placed over the foot while the animal is walking outside and then removed when it is indoors.

Potential complications

- Dyspnoea
- Venous stasis
- Limb oedema
- Moist dermatitis
- Maceration of skin underlying a wet bandage
- Contamination of wounds
- Pressure necrosis

Thoracocentesis – needle

Indications/Use

- Rapid stabilization of acute respiratory distress due to the accumulation of air or fluid in the pleural space
- To obtain samples of pleural fluid for diagnostic evaluation
- See **Thoracostomy tube placement** for alternative techniques to remove a large volume of pleural fluid or very viscous pleural effusions, or where repeated thoracic drainage is required

Contraindications

- Ongoing haemorrhage into the pleural space, e.g. haemothorax due to a coagulopathy or trauma
- Small volume of effusion or air

Equipment

- As for **Aseptic preparation – (a) non-surgical procedures**
- 19–23 G ¾ to 1 inch butterfly needle
  OR an over-the-needle catheter: 18–20 G for medium to large dogs (>10 kg); 20–22 G for cats and small dogs (up to 10 kg)
- 3-way tap
- Fine-bore (2 mm) short extension tubing for use with the over-the-needle catheter. This allows the syringe to move independently from the needle or catheter, reducing the risk of lung laceration and minimizing the risk of dislodging the needle or catheter from its desired position
- 5 ml syringe
- 10–60 ml syringe (depending on the expected volume of air or fluid within the pleural space)
- Measuring container to collect pleural fluid
- Local anaesthetic solution or cream (e.g. EMLA)
- EDTA tube, sterile plain tube, microscope slides

Patient preparation and positioning

- Sedation is often not required, although it may be necessary to prevent movement of the patient during the procedure. Care should be taken when administering sedatives to a dyspnoeic patient.
- Consider the use of supplementary flow-by oxygen; remove the face mask if this distresses the animal.
- Manual restraint in sternal recumbency is usually the easiest position for the animal and the most efficient for drainage. Alternatively, a sitting position or lateral recumbency may be used.
- **Aseptic preparation – (a) non-surgical procedures** should be performed on an area of skin on the lateral thorax, to include skin within a 15 cm radius of the proposed site of thoracocentesis. A skin drape is usually not required.

- Local anaesthetic solution may be instilled into the subcutaneous tissues and muscles at the proposed site. *Alternatively*, if the animal is stable enough to wait, local anaesthetic cream (e.g. EMLA) can be applied over the proposed site 20 minutes in advance of thoracocentesis.

> ### WHICH SIDE?
> - Which side of the animal to use for thoracocentesis is dictated by clinical examination and the results of diagnostic imaging.
> - In some animals, bilateral thoracocentesis may be required, especially when draining bilateral effusions containing dense flocculent material (e.g. pyothorax).

Technique

Thoracocentesis is usually performed at the 7th or 8th intercostal space unless radiography or ultrasonography indicates otherwise. To identify the 7th or 8th intercostal space, count cranially from the most caudal intercostal space which is the 12th.

The site of needle insertion is:

- Half way up the thoracic wall if both pleural air and fluid are present
- In the ventral third of the thorax if only pleural fluid is present
- In the dorsal third of the thorax if only pleural air is present.

Butterfly needle

1 Attach the butterfly needle to a 3-way tap, extension tubing and 5 ml syringe, with the 3-way tap turned so that it is 'off' to the butterfly needle. Hand the 3-way tap, extension tubing and syringe to an assistant.

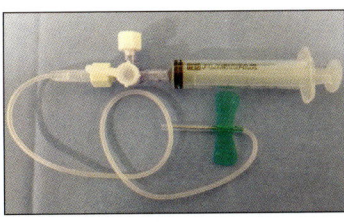

2 Insert the butterfly needle through the skin and intercostal muscle at the cranial border of the rib to avoid the intercostal vessels and nerves (which run along the caudal border of each rib).

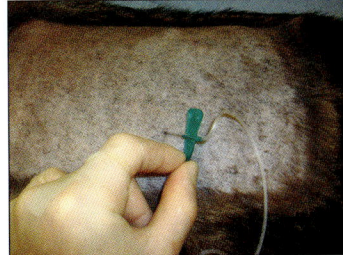

3 Advance the needle slowly into the pleural space. Once the needle is through the skin, the assistant can turn the 3-way tap to the 'on' position and apply slight negative pressure (no more than 1 ml). If air or fluid enters the syringe, the needle is in the pleural space.

4 As soon as the pleural space is entered, direct the tip of the needle to lie parallel to the thoracic wall to minimize the risk of pulmonary lacerations. The needle should be inserted fully to the hub once inside the pleural space.

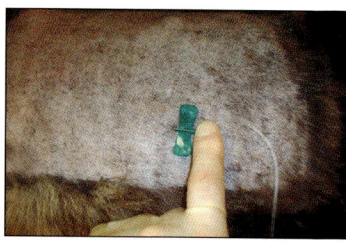

> ### WARNING
>
> - If frank blood is initially aspirated, consider whether this is due to haemothorax or iatrogenic haemorrhage.
> - Stop draining the thorax and assess whether the sample in the syringe clots; if it does, this is probably iatrogenic haemorrhage from an intercostal or pleural vessel. Fluid from a haemothorax would not be expected to clot.
> - Running a manual PCV on the sample and comparing it to the patient's PCV is useful to differentiate whether the fluid is due to a haemothorax or iatrogenic haemorrhage: the PCV of a haemothorax will be the same as or higher than that of the patient's blood, whereas the PCV of fluid due to iatrogenic haemorrhage will be similar to that of the patient's blood.

5 Turn the 3-way tap to the 'off' position, remove the 5 ml syringe, and attach another syringe suitable for the expected volume of air or fluid within the pleural space.

6 Turn the 3-way tap to the 'on' position and drain the pleural space of fluid or air. Excessive negative pressure should be avoided, especially if using a large syringe to drain pleural fluid.

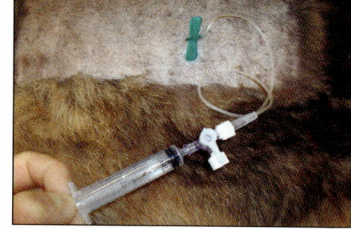

7 Fluid or air can be expelled from the syringe when full, after closing off the 3-way tap to the pleural space. Samples of pleural fluid should be collected into EDTA (for cytology) and sterile plain (for culture) tubes. Fresh air-dried smears of any flocculent material can also be made. Keep a note of how much air or fluid is drained off, i.e. how many syringes are filled.

8 Drainage is complete when no further fluid or air can be drained, or when the veterinary surgeon can feel the lung rubbing against the tip of the needle.

9 The 3-way tap is turned so that it is 'off' to the butterfly needle and the needle is withdrawn from the thorax.

10 Thoracic radiography should be performed after thoracocentesis to look for an initiating cause of a pneumothorax or pleural effusion, and to check for completeness of drainage and complications of the procedure.

Over-the-needle catheter

1 Attach the catheter to a 3-way tap, extension tubing and 5 ml syringe, with the 3-way tap turned so that it is 'off' to the catheter. Hand the 3-way tap, extension tubing and syringe to an assistant.

2 Insert the over-the-needle catheter (cannula and needle) through the skin and intercostal muscle at the cranial border of the rib at the desired intercostal space (see above).

3 Advance the catheter slowly into the pleural space. Once the catheter is through the skin, the assistant can turn the 3-way-tap to the 'on' position and apply slight negative pressure (no more than 1 ml). If air or fluid enters the syringe, the needle is in the pleural space.

4 Once the catheter enters the pleural space, advance the cannula into the thorax over the needle in a caudal direction, so as to direct the tip of the cannula to lie parallel to the thoracic wall. Withdraw the needle and attach the extension tubing with 3-way tap and syringe directly to the catheter. *There is no need to insert the cannula fully into the pleural space.* **See Warning box for Butterfly needle, above.**

5 Continue as points 5 to 10 above.

Potential complications

- Lung laceration
- Pneumothorax
- Iatrogenic infection
- Haemorrhage
- Pulmonary re-expansion injury, leading to the development of pulmonary oedema

FURTHER INFORMATION

For interpretation of the results of fluid analysis, see the *BSAVA Manual of Canine and Feline Clinical Pathology*.

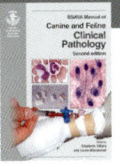

Thoracostomy tube placement – (a) trocar tube

Indications/Use

- Removal of air or fluid from the pleural space when frequent or repeated drainage is expected or required
- Medical management of pyothorax
- Stabilization prior to definitive surgical treatment of pleural space disease
- Removal of air and fluid from the pleural space in the immediate postoperative period following thoracic surgery

> ### WARNINGS
> - There is a risk of injury to thoracic viscera when placing a trocar tube.
> - The use of a small-bore wire-guided thoracostomy tube (see next procedure) should be considered as an alternative, especially when draining air or non- tenacious fluid.
> - However, trocar tubes are particularly useful when draining effusions containing dense flocculent material e.g. pyothorax.

Contraindications

- Severe respiratory compromise: stabilization with oxygen therapy or **thoracocentesis** may be required to improve respiration prior to induction of general anaesthesia
- Severe coagulopathy

Equipment

- As for **Aseptic preparation – (b) non-surgical procedures**
- Silicone or PVC multi-fenestrated trocar thoracostomy tube:
  - Diameter should be approximately the width of the mainstem bronchus as seen on thoracic radiographs (14–16 Fr for cats and tiny dogs; 18–24 Fr for small to medium dogs; 26–36 Fr for large to giant breed dogs)
  - Length should be such that the tip sits at the approximate level of the 2nd rib following placement
- Local anaesthetic solution
- Scalpel
- 3-way tap
- Luer-lock connector
- Intravenous fluid extension tubing
- Atraumatic forceps
- Gate clamp
- 20–50 ml syringe
- Zinc oxide tape
- Measuring container to collect pleural fluid

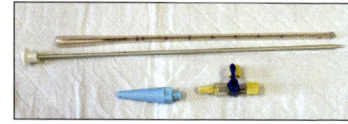

Chest tube with trocar, Luer connector and 3-way tap.

- 0.9% sterile saline or lactated Ringer's solution (Hartmann's)
- Suture material (e.g. 3 metric (2/0 USP) monofilament nylon)
- Light bandage (stockinette, or conforming non-adhesive wrap)
- Elizabethan collar

Patient positioning and preparation

NOTE

Thoracocentesis is not obligatory before placement of a thoracostomy tube. However, careful consideration should be given as to whether drainage would improve the animal's respiratory function so that subsequent general anaesthesia, if required, for tube placement would be safer. If the animal is stable and dyspnoea is not marked, thoracostomy tube placement can proceed without prior drainage. In fact, the presence of air or fluid within the pleural cavity can reduce the chance of iatrogenic lung injury during thoracostomy tube placement. Preoxygenation of the animal for 5 minutes before anaesthesia is strongly recommended.

- General anaesthesia is recommended, although in some animals heavy sedation may be sufficient.
- Local anaesthetic solution should be applied as a bleb to the skin at the site where the drain is to enter.
- Local anaesthetic solution should also be infiltrated into the subcutaneous tissues, intercostal musculature and pleura at a site two intercostal spaces cranial to this point (see below). Consider the use of a long-acting local anaesthetic (see **Local anaesthesia**), to provide analgesia in the post-procedure period.

NERVE BLOCK

An intercostal nerve block can be administered at the proposed intercostal space of entry and 2–3 intercostal spaces cranial and caudal to this.

- The intercostal nerves run just caudal to the ribs in a dorsoventral direction.
- Local anaesthetic solution should be applied as far dorsal as possible in the tissues caudal to each rib.
- After needle insertion, draw back on the syringe to ensure that the needle is not within a blood vessel prior to anaesthetic injection.

- **Aseptic preparation – (b) non-surgical procedures** of the lateral thorax should be performed, to include an area craniocaudally from the caudal border of the scapula to just caudal to the last rib, and dorsoventrally from the vertebrae to the sternum.

WHICH SIDE?

- Which side of the animal to use for placement of the thoracostomy tube is dictated by clinical examination and the results of diagnostic imaging.
- In some animals, bilateral thoracostomy tubes may be required, especially when draining bilateral effusions containing dense flocculent material (e.g. pyothorax).

- The animal should be maintained in sternal recumbency during preparation, but thoracic drain insertion is most easily performed with the animal in lateral recumbency.

Technique

1 Make a small skin incision using a scalpel at the junction of the dorsal to middle third of the thorax at the 10th intercostal space.

2 Insert the thoracostomy tube with the trocar into the skin incision and under the skin. Advance it in a cranial and slightly ventral direction to approximately the 8th intercostal space. This creates a subcutaneous tunnel to prevent air tracking from the environment along the tube and into the thorax.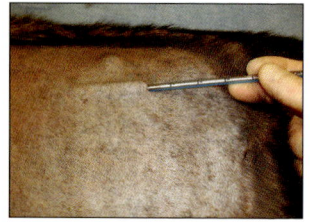

Alternatively, an assistant can grasp the skin over the lateral thorax at approximately the 4th rib and pull the skin incision site cranially to the level of the 8th intercostal space; the assistant then keeps the skin in that position. This avoids the need to tunnel the thoracostomy tube under the skin.

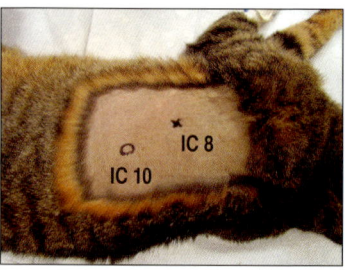
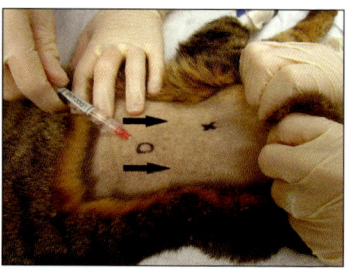

ALTERNATIVE SUBCUTANEOUS TUNNEL TECHNIQUE

Placement of the thoracostomy tube under the latissimus dorsi muscle may create a better seal around the tube:

i.   Make the initial skin incision directly over a rib.
ii. Tunnel the trocar tip of the thoracostomy tube on to the underling rib so that the trocar tip perforates the latissimus dorsi muscle.
iii. Direct the drain cranially between the rib and the overlying latissimus dorsi muscle.

3   Hold the thoracostomy tube and trocar perpendicular to the 8th intercostal space and introduce it into the thorax by means of a short, controlled push with the heel of the hand. **Hold the drain firmly close to the tip with the other hand to prevent excessive and uncontrolled entry into the thorax.**

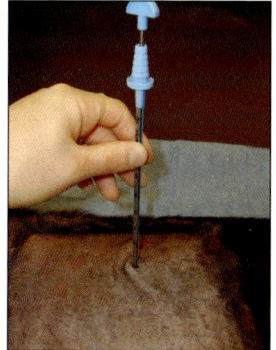

4   Once the thoracostomy tube has entered the thoracic cavity, angle it so that the tip points cranially and ventrally.

5   Advance the thoracostomy tube over the trocar in a cranioventral direction, to approximately the level of the 2nd rib.

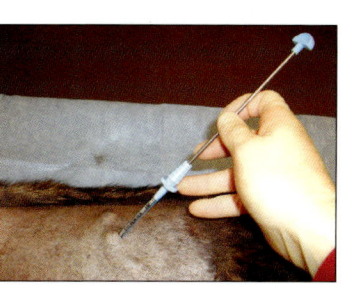

> **NOTE**
>
> The cranial end of the thoracostomy tube should ideally lie in the ventral thorax, before the sternum begins to rise towards the thoracic inlet; the tip of the tube should curve gently upwards. This tube location should enable both fluid and air to be drained. However, this exact position is not always possible.

6   If applicable, the assistant now releases the skin and it retracts caudally, forming a valve-like seal between the skin entry site and where the tube passes though the intercostal muscles.

7   Remove the trocar and immediately occlude the tube temporarily with atraumatic forceps, whilst pre-placing a gate clamp on the tube and attaching a Luer-lock connector and 3-way tap.

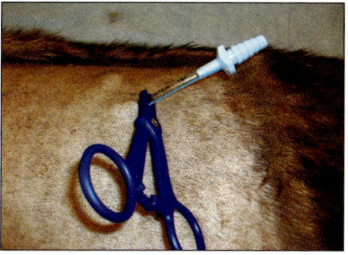

8   Remove the forceps, enabling drainage of the thorax using a syringe attached to the 3-way tap (see below).

9   Secure the thoracostomy tube to the thoracic wall by means of a Chinese finger-trap suture.

10 Radiography should be performed at this point to confirm correct positioning within the thorax, to look for an initiating cause, and to check for complications.

11 The tube should be further secured by applying a butterfly tab of zinc oxide tape and suturing this to the patient.

12 Place a sterile dressing over the site of thoracic drain insertion. Cover with a light bandage.

13 Place an Elizabethan collar to prevent interference with the tube and possible pneumothorax.

Drainage

- The thorax is drained either by intermittent suction using a syringe applied directly to the 3-way tap, or via intravenous fluid extension tubing.
- The latter is preferable in restless or uncooperative patients, as there is no direct manipulation of the chest tube while drainage or lavage is being performed.
- Excessive negative pressure (>5 ml) should not be applied to the syringe, as this can result in damage to structures within the pleural cavity.
- Initial drainage is performed every 4 hours, but the frequency can be altered subsequently depending on the volume of fluid or air removed.
- In animals with persistent, high-volume pneumothorax, consider the use of continuous suction drainage or the use of a one-way valve such as the Heimlich valve.
- In an animal with a pyothorax, twice-daily lavage should be performed using warmed 0.9% sterile saline or lactated Ringer's solution (Hartmann's). Infuse approximately 10–20 ml/kg of fluid aseptically over 5–10 minutes, while monitoring respiration. At least 75% of the fluid should be recovered; altering the animal's position and then re-aspirating after a few minutes may help fluid retrieval.
- As a general rule, thoracic drainage is continued until the volume of fluid or air reduces to <2 ml/kg/day.

Tube care and maintenance

- Animals with thoracostomy tubes in place should have *constant*, ideally continuous, supervision: to ensure security of the tube connections; to observe for changes in respiratory rate and effort; and to prevent self-interference with the drain.
- The dressing and bandage must be changed and all connections checked *at least once a day*. Thoracic drains should be handled in an *aseptic* fashion during bandage changes and drainage of the pleural cavity.
- A non-functional thoracostomy tube should be removed promptly. This can usually be done without sedation by cutting the anchoring suture material and removing the tube in one smooth motion. The skin incision site can usually be left to heal by secondary intention, although if a large hole exists, consider the use a single suture or tissue glue.

Potential complications

- Lung laceration
- Iatrogenic infection
- A small-volume iatrogenic pneumothorax may occur at the time of catheter placement; a larger pneumothorax may develop if the tube becomes dislodged
- Haemorrhage
- Pulmonary re-expansion injury, leading to the development of pulmonary oedema
- Accidental removal of the tube
- Collapse of the tube due to excess suction pressure
- Obstruction of the tube with tenacious fluid or as a result of kinking of the drain

Thoracostomy tube placement – (b) small-bore wire-guided

Photos from *BSAVA Manual of Feline Practice* and courtesy of Dan Lewis

Indications/Use

- As for **Thoracostomy tube placement – (a) trocar tube**

> **OPTIONS**
>
> - Small-bore wire-guided thoracostomy tubes are reported to be associated with fewer complications compared with large-bore trocar tubes, are easier to place and are more comfortable for the patient.
> - However, it may be difficult to drain effusions containing dense flocculent material (e.g. pyothorax) with a small-bore wire-guided tube. In this situation, **Thoracostomy tube placement – (a) trocar tube** is advised.

Contraindications

- As for **Thoracostomy tube placement – (a) trocar tube**

Equipment

- As for **Aseptic preparation – (a) non-surgical procedures**
- A proprietary small-bore-wire-guided kit in a sterile pack containing:
    - 14 G, 20 cm long radiopaque polyurethane catheter (thoracostomy tube) with a multi-fenestrated tip and suture wing to facilitate attachment to skin
    - 14 G (green, used in cats) and 18 G (orange, used in dogs) over-the-needle catheter introducers
    - 60 cm 'J-tip' guidewire coiled up in a protective sheathing with 'thumb-wheel' adaptor for ease of introduction
    - Needle-free drainage cap
    - Extra suture wings and locking covers

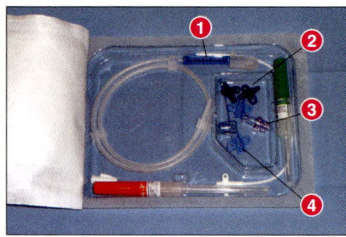

1 = 'Thumb-wheel' adapter for wire introduction. 2 = Extra suture wings. 3 = Needle-free drainage cap. 4 = Locking cover for extra suture wing.

- Local anaesthetic solution
- Scalpel
- 20–50 ml syringe
- 3-way tap
- Intravenous fluid extension tubing
- 0.9% sterile saline or lactated Ringer's solution (Hartmann's)
- Measuring container to collect pleural fluid
- Suture material (e.g. 3 metric (2/0 USP) monofilament non-absorbable)
- Light bandage (stockinette, or conforming non-adhesive wrap)
- Elizabethan collar

Patient positioning and preparation

> **NOTE**
>
> Thoracocentesis is not obligatory before placement of a thoracostomy tube. However, careful consideration should be given as to whether drainage would improve the animal's respiratory function so that subsequent general anaesthesia, if required, for tube placement would be safer. If the animal is stable and dyspnoea is not marked, thoracostomy tube placement can proceed without prior drainage. In fact, the presence of air or fluid within the pleural cavity can reduce the chance of iatrogenic lung injury during thoracostomy tube placement. Preoxygenation of the animal for 5 minutes before anaesthesia is strongly recommended.

- Heavy sedation is usually sufficient, although general anaesthesia may be employed if required for additional procedures.
- Local anaesthetic solution should be applied as a bleb to the skin at the proposed site of drain placement. Local anaesthetic solution can also be infiltrated into the subcutaneous tissues, intercostal musculature and pleura. Consider the use of a long-acting local anaesthetic (see **Local anaesthesia**) to provide analgesia in the post-procedure period.
- **Aseptic preparation – (a) non-surgical procedures** of the lateral thorax is required, to include an area at least 15 cm around the proposed site of catheter insertion.

> ### WHICH SIDE?
>
> - Which side of the animal to use for placement of the thoracostomy tube is dictated by clinical examination and the results of diagnostic imaging.
> - In some animals, bilateral thoracostomy tubes may be required, especially when draining bilateral effusions containing dense flocculent material (e.g. pyothorax).

- A fenestrated drape should be centred over the proposed site of catheter insertion – towel clips are not recommended in unanaesthetized patients.
- The catheter can be placed with the animal in sternal or lateral recumbency depending on the preference of the veterinary surgeon.

Technique

1   Prepare the J-wire for insertion by withdrawing it until its tip is just visible outside the 'thumb-wheel' adaptor.

2   Make a small stab skin incision, using a scalpel, over the 7th or 8th intercostal space at the junction of the dorsal to middle third of the thorax.

3   Insert the over-the-needle catheter introducer through the stab incision and into the thoracic cavity. The catheter introducer should enter the thorax over the cranial border of the rib to avoid the intercostal vessels and nerves which run along the caudal aspect of each rib.

   Alternatively, the stab incision can be made at the 9th intercostal space, and the over-the-needle catheter introducer tunnelled subcutaneously and cranially over one to two intercostal spaces. This step further reduces the risk of air gaining access to the thorax around the thoracostomy tube or if the tube is accidentally removed. However, due to the small diameter of the tube, this step is usually unnecessary.

4   Once the introducer enters the pleural cavity, advance the catheter introducer fully over the needle stylet.

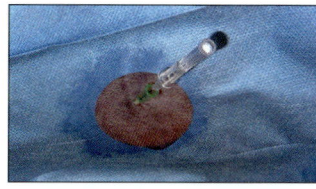

5   Remove the needle stylet.

6   Using the 'thumb-wheel' adaptor, thread the previously prepared guidewire out of the protective sheathing through the introducer catheter and into the thorax. Advance the guidewire in a cranioventral direction by approximately 10–20 cm or until resistance is encountered. **The guidewire should be held at all times when it is partially within the thorax.**

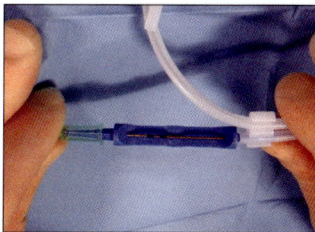

7   Remove the catheter introducer from the thorax by threading it off the guidewire, leaving only the guidewire within the thorax.

8   Pre-measure the polyurethane catheter (thoracostomy tube) and advance it over the guidewire into the thoracic cavity. The distance from the most distal side hole is marked on the catheter.

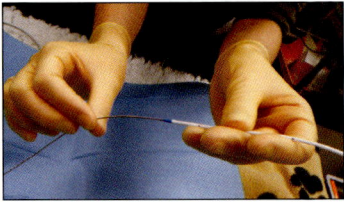

> **NOTE**
>
> The cranial end of the thoracostomy tube should ideally lie in the ventral thorax, before the sternum begins to rise towards the thoracic inlet, and the tip of the tube should curve gently upwards. This tube location should enable both fluid and air to be drained. However, this exact position is not always possible.

9   Once in place remove the guidewire and immediately attach the needle-free drainage cap. Attach a 3-way tap and confirm correct placement by connecting a syringe and attempting drainage.

10 Secure the thoracostomy tube to the skin, using suture material passed through the holes in the suture wing.

11 Radiography should be performed at this point to confirm correct positioning within the thorax, to look

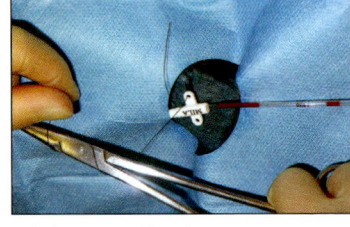

for an initiating cause and to check for complications.

12 Attach additional suture wings to the drain and secure them in place at the proximal end of the drain if it is not fully inserted.

13 Place a sterile dressing over the site of thoracic drain insertion. Cover with a light bandage.

14 Place an Elizabethan collar to prevent interference with the tube and possible pneumothorax.

Drainage

- As for **Thoracostomy tube placement – (a) trocar tube**

Tube care and maintenance

- As for **Thoracostomy tube placement – (a) trocar tube**

Potential complications

- As for **Thoracostomy tube placement – (a) trocar tube**, although small-bore wire-guided tubes are generally associated with fewer complications

Tissue biopsy – needle core

Indications/Use
- To obtain samples from:
    - Superficial masses that can be palpated well enough to be stabilized
    - Masses or organs within a body cavity, usually under ultrasound guidance
- As an alternative to **fine needle aspiration**

Contraindications
- Coagulopathy
- Inability to stabilize or visualize the tissue to be sampled

Equipment
- As for **Aseptic preparation – (a) non-surgical procedures**
- Core biopsy needle: from 14 G (large dogs) to 20 G (cats)
- Local anaesthetic solution
- No. 11 or 15 scalpel
- Container with 10% neutral buffered formalin
- Suture materials or tissue glue
- Ultrasound machine

Patient preparation and positioning
- The procedure can usually be performed under heavy sedation.
- Deeper, ultrasound-guided procedures will normally require general anaesthesia.
- If the mass to be sampled is superficial, local anaesthetic solution is infiltrated into the surrounding area.
- The patient is positioned to allow optimal stabilization or visualization (if under ultrasound guidance) of the mass.
- **Aseptic preparation – (a) non-surgical procedures** of an area several centimetres wide, centred on the needle entry point, is required.

> **NOTES**
>
> - When sampling vascular organs, especially the liver, haemostasis needs to be checked by way of measurement of prothrombin time, activated partial thromboplastin time and a **platelet count**.
> - The clinician also needs to ensure that the approach to the mass or organ will not result in perforation of vessels, the biliary, urinary or gastrointestinal tract.
> - It should be remembered that there is still a risk of haemorrhage despite normal coagulation, and it is important to have the option of prompt surgical intervention in case of complications.
> - The animal also needs to be kept under close observation *after* the procedure and monitored for evidence of haemorrhage (e.g. tachycardia, pallor, weakness, reduced pulse quality).

Technique

1 Make a small stab incision through the skin, using a scalpel blade.

2 Prior to insertion, prepare the biopsy needle by pulling back on the plunger until a firm click is felt, indicating that the needle spring is locked into a ready position.

3 With the stylet fully retracted, so that the specimen notch is completely covered by the cutting cannula, advance the needle into the tissue to be sampled.

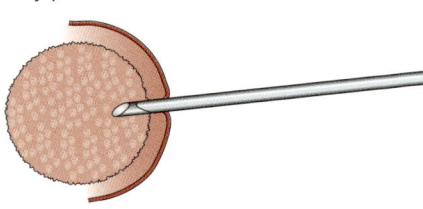

4 Advance the stylet with the thumb to expose the specimen notch within the tissue to be sampled.

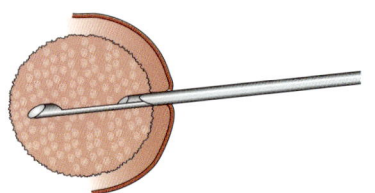

5 Rotate to and fro to ensure that tissue fills the biopsy notch.

6 Fire the cutting cannula by fully depressing the plunger.

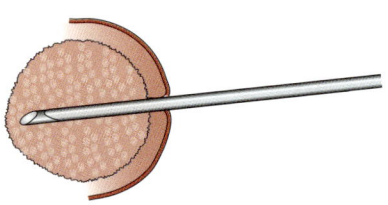

7 Withdraw the biopsy needle.

8 To remove the tissue specimen, pull back on the plunger until a firm click is felt. Push the stylet forward to expose the tissue specimen within the notch.

9 Gently remove the sample with a fine hypodermic needle, or by irrigation with saline into the fixative.

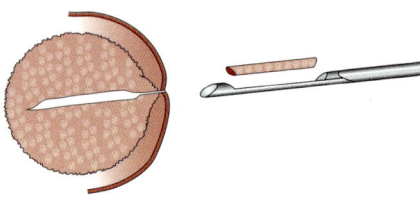

10 Leave the skin incision to heal, or close with a single suture or tissue adhesive.

Sample handling

- Fix solid tissue samples in 10% neutral buffered formalin solution.
- Impression smears or squash smears (see **Fine needle aspiration**) of tissue samples can also be made.

Potential complications

- Haemorrhage. Sampling of vascular organs such as the liver, spleen or kidneys should be preceded by an assessment of coagulation status; the patient should also be monitored for several hours after the procedure
- Damage to internal viscera

Tracheostomy

Indications/Use

- Management of upper airway obstruction that is non-responsive to medical management
- Maintenance of prolonged mechanical ventilation
- Anaesthesia for certain surgeries of the upper airway and pharynx, where an endotracheal (ET) tube would limit surgical access

> **WARNING**
>
> - **Tracheostomy tube placement in a dyspnoeic patient with upper airway obstruction in an emergency situation, by an *inexperienced* veterinary surgeon may not result in optimal results.**
> - **Stabilization with oxygen therapy, sedatives, emergency anaesthesia and endotracheal intubation, *prior* to tracheostomy tube placement may lead to better results.**

Equipment

- As for **Aseptic preparation – (b) surgical procedures**
- Tracheostomy tubes:
    - Routine airway maintenance: non-cuffed tracheostomy tube with an inner cannula; outer diameter no more than 75% of the luminal diameter of the trachea
    - Maintenance of anaesthesia or prolonged mechanical ventilation: tracheostomy tube with an inner cannula and a high-volume low-pressure cuff

> **NOTE**
>
> Small tracheostomy tubes suitable for dogs <10 kg and for cats are not generally available with an inner cannula.

- Suture materials
- Nylon tape (usually supplied with the tracheostomy tube)
- Range of narrow ET tubes and stylet for endotracheal intubation
- Soft tissue surgical instrument set

Patient preparation and positioning

- Where possible, tracheostomy tubes should be placed under general anaesthesia in a controlled environment.
- This most often means placement of an ET tube prior to tracheostomy tube placement. Failure to achieve endotracheal intubation will necessitate immediate tracheal intubation following anaesthetic induction: be prepared to use a stylet to achieve placement of a standard ET tube or a dog urinary catheter instead of an ET tube in cases of severe upper airway obstruction.
- The animal should be placed in dorsal recumbency. The neck should be supported in extension by placement of a sandbag underneath it. The forelegs should be pulled caudally and secured on either side of the thorax.
- **Aseptic preparation – (b) surgical procedures** of the ventral neck.

Technique

1   Palpate the larynx and trachea and make an approximately 7 cm (length depends on the size of the animal) midline skin incision, running caudally from the larynx.

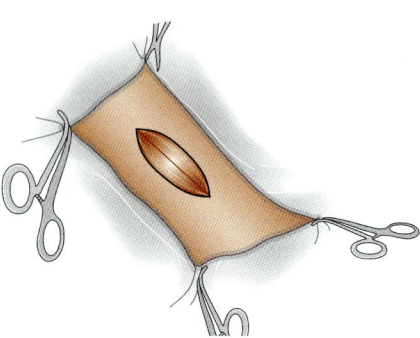

2   Separate the sternohyoideus muscles at the midline and retract them laterally to visualize the trachea. The caudal thyroid vein, with small branches on either side, runs along the midline in the fascia between the sternohydoideus muscles. Try to preserve this vessel to avoid unnecessary haemorrhage.

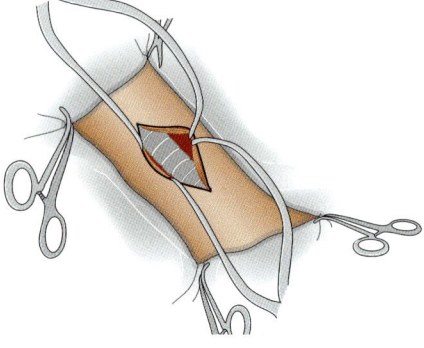

3 Place stay sutures around the tracheal rings just cranial and caudal to the proposed annular ligament incision. These stay sutures allow for stabilization of the trachea when inserting or changing the tracheostomy tube.

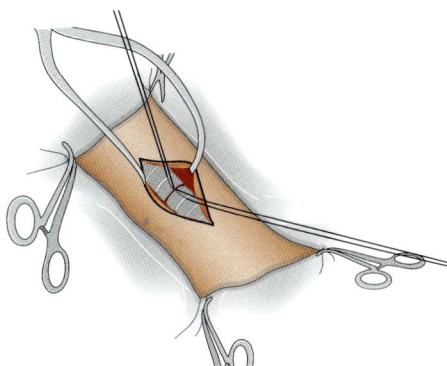

4 Make an incision in one of the annular ligaments between the 3rd and 5th tracheal rings. The incision of the annular ligament should not extend more than 50–60% of the diameter of the trachea. The recurrent laryngeal nerves, which look like fine white threads, run laterally either side of the trachea and should be avoided.

5 Insert the tracheostomy tube into the trachea, using the round tipped inner stylet provided. Withdraw the stylet. Insert inner hollow cannula (where available).

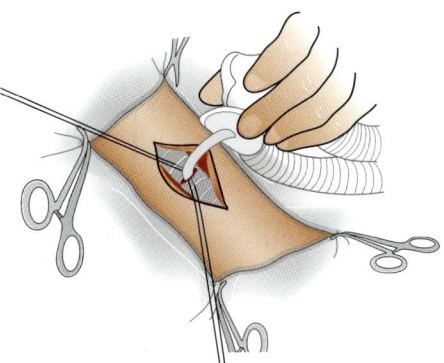

6 Appose the skin cranial and caudal to the tube with simple interrupted sutures, allowing a large enough opening for re-placement of the tracheostomy tube into the trachea if necessary.

7 Secure the tracheostomy tube around the neck with nylon tape.

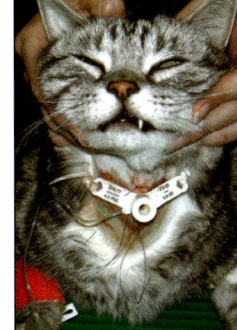

> **NOTE**
>
> Note that the stay sutures remain around the tracheal rings for postoperative care.

(Photo courtesy of Dan Brockman)

Tracheostomy tube care

- 24-hour-care is essential to prevent potentially fatal occlusion of the tube by exudates and airway mucus, and to detect tube dislodgement.
- The inner cannula should be removed for cleaning whenever an increased noise or effort associated with breathing is noticed, or every 2 hours initially. The cannula should be cleaned thoroughly using warm water, dried by evaporation and re-placed.
- For tracheostomy tubes without an inner cannula, the entire tube should be removed for cleaning. Ideally, a spare tracheostomy tube should be available for immediate placement into the trachea following removal of the dirty tracheostomy tube. The stay sutures placed around the tracheal rings above and below the tracheostomy site should be used to gently bring the trachea to the level of the skin and to open the trachea.
- Humidification: if the inner cannula is repeatedly full of tenacious mucus and exudate, either nebulized air should be provided for periods for the animal to breathe, or 0.1 ml/kg sterile saline should be instilled into the tube every 2 hours (the latter may induce transient coughing).
- Suction: this is not a benign procedure and should be performed *only as required*. It is more commonly needed in smaller dogs and cats. The patient should be pre-oxygenated for approximately 10 breaths. A sterile suction catheter should be introduced aseptically into the tracheostomy tube and suction applied for *no more than 15 seconds,* while gently rotating the suction tube. The suction catheter should remain within the tube during suctioning and only be inserted into the vulnerable trachea if absolutely necessary to clear an obstruction distal to the tracheostomy tube.
- The tracheostomy wound should be inspected daily and cleaned with sterile saline-soaked swabs as necessary.
- If the above measures do not relieve breathing difficulty, the whole tube should be changed. This should *not* be done in the absence of a veterinary surgeon or facilities for endotracheal intubation and administration of oxygen. The patient is pre-oxygenated and the trachea stabilized using the stay sutures placed around the tracheal rings above and below the tracheostomy site. The old tube is removed and a new one inserted rapidly.

Potential complications

- Tracheostomy site dermatitis and infection
- Obstruction of the tracheostomy tube
- Tracheostomy tube dislodgement
- Obstruction of the trachea distal to the tracheostomy tube
- Haemorrhage around the tracheostomy site
- Pressure necrosis of the trachea
- Pneumonia
- Damage to the recurrent laryngeal nerves resulting in unilateral or bilateral laryngeal paralysis
- Fatal airway obstruction

Transtracheal wash

Indications/Use

- To obtain a sample for cytology and bacteriology from the airways of medium and large-sized dogs
- Can be used where general anaesthesia is a risk to the patient
- Generally yields samples representative of the trachea and primary or (at best) secondary bronchi, although some material from the lower bronchioles and alveoli may be collected
- The upper airway of dogs and cats may also be sampled by **endotracheal wash**
- The lower airways of dogs and cats may be sampled by **bronchoalveolar lavage**

Contraindications

- Compromised respiratory function
- Animals with pulmonary parenchymal disease, rather than tracheal or bronchial disease

Equipment

- As for **Aseptic preparation – (a) non-surgical procedures**
- Through-the-needle long jugular catheter (19–22 G, 8 inches long for medium (<20 kg) dogs; 19 G, 12 or 24 inches long for larger dogs)
  OR 12–14 G over-the-needle catheter and male dog urinary catheter (3–6 Fr). Check that the urinary catheter passes easily through the over-the-needle catheter before starting. The tip of the catheter can be cut off to remove the side holes, but care must be taken to ensure that the tip is not sharp
- Local anaesthetic solution
- 2 ml syringe and 21 G hypodermic needle
- No. 11 or 15 scalpel
- 500 ml bag of warm 0.9% sterile saline
- 10 ml and 20 ml syringes
- Sterile plain and EDTA collection tubes
- Microscope slides
- Dressing materials

Patient preparation and positioning

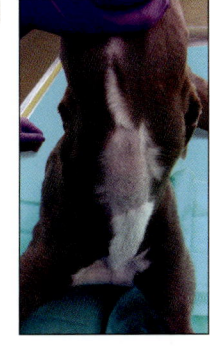

- The procedure can usually be performed without sedation unless the animal is fractious. If sedation is used, ideally the animal should be awake enough to cough.
- The patient is positioned standing or sitting at the edge of a table or on the floor, with its nose elevated and its feet restrained.
- **Aseptic preparation – (a) non-surgical procedures** of the skin of the ventral neck from just above to several centimetres below the larynx is required.

Technique

1 The site of catheter placement is ideally through the cricothyroid ligament, although a site between tracheal rings 2 to 5 distal to the larynx can also be used. At the most cranial end of the trachea, a wide ring is palpated that protrudes more than the tracheal rings, and this is the cricoid cartilage. The cricothyroid ligament is the small triangular membrane just cranial to the cricoid cartilage. In smaller dogs the only palpable landmark may be the cricoid cartilage and so the needle is inserted just cranial to this larger ring.

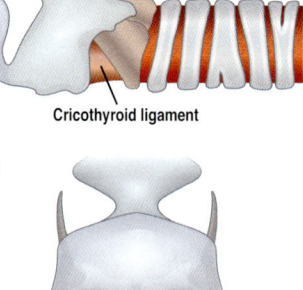

Cricothyroid ligament

Cricothyroid ligament

2 Infiltrate 0.5–1 ml of local anaesthetic solution into the skin and subcutis over this area.

3 Stabilize the larynx between the thumb and forefinger, and make a small skin incision through the skin over the site of entry.

4 ***Over-the-needle catheter:***

   i Push the over-the-needle catheter through the cricothyroid ligament or between two tracheal rings, with the bevel of the needle facing down. Firm pressure is required to achieve this.

   ii Once the needle is in the lumen of the trachea, the needle can be removed, leaving only the catheter.

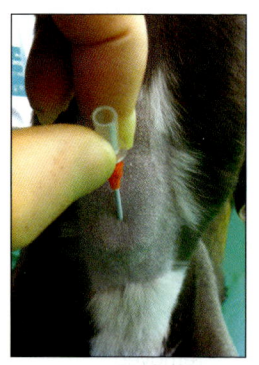

   iii Thread the male dog urinary catheter through the over-the-needle catheter, ideally to the level of the carina (approximately the 4th intercostal space) or, if not, as far down as it will pass.

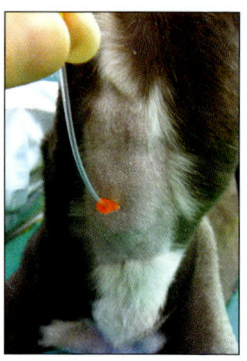

iv Instil approximately 0.5 ml/kg warm sterile saline through the urinary catheter.

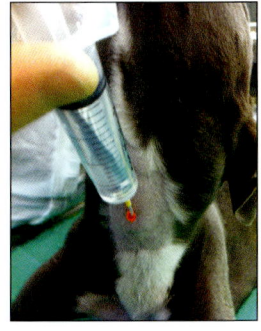

Through-the-needle catheter:

i Push the needle through the cricothyroid ligament or between two tracheal rings, with the bevel of the needle facing down. Firm pressure if required to achieve this.

ii Advance the needle approximately 1–2 cm into the trachea after the lumen is entered. Angle the needle at approximately 45 degrees to direct it down the tracheal lumen.

iii Pass the catheter through the needle, ideally to the level of the carina (approximately the 4th intercostal space) or, if not, as far down as it will pass. The animal may cough at this point. If the catheter does not feed easily, back the needle out of the trachea a short distance, as the tip of the needle may be pressed up against the wall of the trachea.

iv Once the full length of the catheter is in the trachea, withdraw the needle and inject approximately 0.5 ml/kg warm sterile saline into the catheter.

5 **Immediately** aspirate back the material using a 10 or 20 ml syringe.

6 Repeat the injection of saline and aspiration two to three times if required.

7 Remove the catheter and apply pressure to the region for 2 minutes before covering in a temporary light dressing. This dressing can be removed after 1–2 hours.

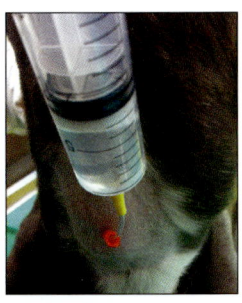

NOTES

- A total recovery of 1–3 ml of a slightly turbid fluid with a foamy layer at the top (representative of surfactant) represents a good sample.
- The optimal recovery is often during patient coughing; coupage and turning the patient may also improve the yield.
- If nothing is recovered, lay the animal in sternal recumbency (if sitting) with the nose, head and neck in a more neutral position and repeat the flush.

Sample handling

- Submit an aliquot of the sample in a sterile plain tube for culture.
- Place an aliquot in an EDTA tube for cytology.
- The cells collected are fragile, so samples should be processed as soon as possible. If samples are to be sent to an external laboratory, fresh air-dried unstained smears of any flocculent/mucoid material should also be made (see **Fine needle aspiration**). Direct smears of the fluid can also be made, but most samples are poorly cellular.

Potential complications

- Larynx or airway spasm
- Subcutaneous emphysema
- Pneumomediastinum
- Infection at the needle site
- Catheter breakage and aspiration of the catheter into the airway
- Worsening of respiratory status due to stress of the procedure

FURTHER INFORMATION

Details on cytology of upper respiratory tract samples can be found in the *BSAVA Manual of Canine and Feline Clinical Pathology.*

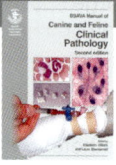

Urethral catheterization – (a) male dog

Indications/Use

- To collect urine for **urinalysis**
- To empty the urinary bladder
- To administer radiographic contrast media into the lower urinary tract (see **Retrograde urethrography/vaginourethrography**)
- An **indwelling** urinary catheter is indicated:
  - To maintain constant, controlled bladder drainage
  - To maintain a patent urethra
  - To monitor urine output
  - To assist with nursing care of the recumbent patient and of the patient that is unable to urinate voluntarily

Contraindications

- Pre-existing urethral trauma
- Large space-occupying urethral mass or urethral stricture
- Urine collected by catheterization is *not* optimal for microbiology, as the sample may be contaminated. **Cystocentesis** is preferred

Equipment

- Catheters

Catheter type	Material	Indwelling?	Sizes (Fr)	Length (cm)
Dog catheter	Flexible nylon (polyamide)	No	6–10	50–60
Silicone Foley	Flexible medical grade silicone	Yes	5–10	30, 55

- Sterile soft gauze swabs
- Antiseptic solution: 4% chlorhexidine gluconate or 10% povidone–iodine
- Gloves
- Sterile aqueous lubricant, e.g. K-Y jelly
- Plain sample pot
- Kidney dish
- 5–10 ml syringe

If the catheter is to be indwelling:
- For silicone Foley catheters, water sufficient to fill balloon
- For standard flexible nylon (polyamide) catheters: suture materials; zinc oxide tape
- Sterile intravenous fluid administration set and empty fluid bag or commercial closed urine collection system, with appropriate adapters for attachment to selected urinary catheter
- Elizabethan collar

Patient preparation and positioning

- Male dogs will generally allow urethral catheterization under gentle physical restraint.
- Sedation may be required for fractious patients.
- General anaesthesia may be required for humane reasons, e.g. patient with fractured pelvis.
- The patient should be restrained in lateral recumbency, with the upper leg held away from the prepuce.
- The prepuce should be cleaned with the antiseptic solution, using swabs or a syringe.
- The area around the prepuce can be clipped, especially in long-haired breeds.

Technique

1 Remove the catheter from the outer wrapper and cut a feeding sleeve from the inner sterile packaging, to allow easy feeding of the catheter into the urethra using a 'no touch' technique. If using a silicone Foley catheter, feed the guide wire up the centre of the catheter.
2 An assistant should grasp the caudal os penis with one hand and retract the prepuce caudally with the other hand, exposing the glans penis.
3 Lubricate the catheter and insert the tip into the urethra.
4 Advance the catheter into the urethra. Resistance may be met: at the os penis, where there is a slight narrowing of the urethra; at the ischial arch; and at the prostate, if enlarged.
5 Once the catheter is inserted to the level of the caudal os penis, the grip on the penis is relaxed to allow further unobstructed passage of the catheter. Angling the penis caudally may straighten the urethra to ease passage. Steady but gentle pressure should overcome any resistance. If the catheter cannot be passed, re-evaluate the catheter size.
6 When the catheter tip enters the bladder and urine appears in the catheter hub, continue to advance an additional 2 cm to ensure adequate length beyond the trigone.
7 If using a silicone Foley catheter, inflate the balloon with water once the tip of the catheter is in the bladder.
8 Proceed according to reason for catheterization (e.g. drain bladder, collect urine sample, administer contrast agent).

Sample handling

- For **urinalysis**:
  - Approximately 5 ml is required
  - Samples should be collected into a plain tube.

Indwelling catheters

CATHETER CHOICE
A silicone Foley catheter is preferred for indwelling use.

1   Attach a sterile intravenous administration set and empty fluid bag
    to the urinary catheter and maintain as a closed collection system.
    Alternatively, attach a commercial sterile closed collection urine
    bag to the catheter: a catheter adapter may be required.
2   Place an Elizabethan collar.

Potential complications

- Trauma to the urethra or urinary bladder
- Iatrogenic urinary tract infection

Urethral catheterization – (b) bitch

Indications/Use

As for **Urethral catheterization – (a) male dog**

Contraindications

As for **Urethral catheterization – (a) male dog**

Equipment

- Catheters

Catheter type	Material	Indwelling?	Sizes (Fr)	Length (cm)
Dog catheter	Flexible nylon (polyamide)	No	6–10	50–60
Foley	Flexible medical-grade silicone	Yes	5–10	30, 55
	Teflon-coated latex	Yes	8–16	30–40

- Sterile vaginal speculum and light source
- Sterile soft gauze swabs
- 4% chlorhexidine gluconate or 10% povidone–iodine
- Sterile gloves
- Sterile aqueous lubricant, e.g. K-Y jelly
- Plain sample pot
- Kidney dish
- 5–10 ml syringe

If the catheter is to be made indwelling:

- For Foley catheter: water sufficient to fill balloon; guidewire
- For standard flexible nylon (polyamide) catheter: suture materials; zinc oxide tape
- Sterile intravenous fluid administration set and empty fluid bag or commercial closed urine collection system, with appropriate adapters for attachment to selected urinary catheter
- Elizabethan collar

Patient preparation and positioning

- Bitches may require sedation.
- General anaesthesia may be required for humane reasons, e.g. patient with fractured pelvis.
- The patient may be positioned:
  - In dorsal recumbency with the hindlimbs held cranially (ideally, or in a frogleg position) (for direct visualization)
  - In lateral recumbency (right lateral recumbency for a right-handed operator; left lateral recumbency for a left-handed operator) (for digital palpation)
  - In sternal recumbency with the hindlimbs over the edge of the table (for direct visualization or digital palpation).
- Clean the vulva with the antiseptic to remove any discharge and surface dirt.

Technique

Direct visualization of urethral orifice

Photos courtesy of Amanda Boag

1 If using a dog catheter, remove it from its outer wrapping and expose the *tip only* from the inner sleeve.
2 If using a Foley catheter, remove it completely from its packaging. Handle the catheter with sterile gloves. Insert a guide wire into the catheter tip to stiffen it.
3 Insert a speculum into the vestibule, taking care not to enter the ventrally placed clitoral fossa. The slit of the speculum should be positioned ventrally, allowing the raised external urethral orifice to be identified on the floor (ventral) of the cranial vestibule. Visualization of the 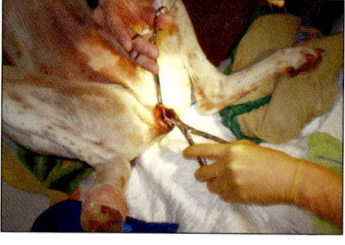 external urethral orifice is often made easier if an assistant pulls on the ventral vulva lips to straighten the vestibule.
4 Lubricate the tip of the catheter and insert it into the urethral orifice under direct visualization.
5 Advance the catheter along the urethra and into the bladder.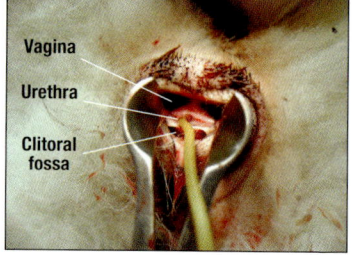
6 If using a Foley catheter, it may be advantageous to insert the catheter all the way into the bladder with the guide wire still in place. Remove the guide wire and inflate the balloon once the tip of the catheter is in the bladder.
7 Proceed according to reason for catheterization (e.g. drain bladder, collect urine sample, administer contrast agent).

Digital palpation of urethral orifice

If a vaginal speculum is not available the catheter can be inserted 'blindly', using digital palpation of the urethral papilla.

> **GLOVES**
>
> Sterile gloves are recommended to prevent iatrogenic urinary tract infection.

1 If using a dog catheter, remove the catheter from its outer wrapping and the inner package in an aseptic fashion.

2 If using a Foley catheter, a guide wire may be used but is not usually required.

3 Place sterile water-soluble lubricant on the catheter and on your index finger.

4 Place this finger into the vestibule and, while gently applying pressure on its floor, move the finger cranially. The urethral papilla is palpated as a slit on a slight 'bulge' of mucosa.

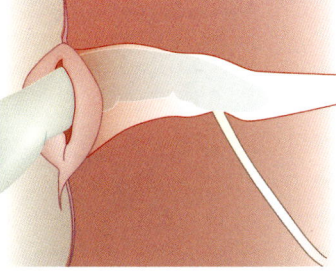

5 While applying gentle pressure over the papilla, feed the catheter under the finger and guide it into the urethra with your other hand. If the orifice is missed, the catheter will run past the fingertip. *Alternatively*, especially in small animals, the urethral orifice can be palpated and the catheter fed into the orifice using the same index finger.

6 If using a Foley catheter, inflate the balloon once the tip of the catheter is in the bladder.

7 Proceed according to reason for catheterization (e.g. drain bladder, collect urine sample, administer contrast agent).

Sample handling

■ For **urinalysis**:
  ▪ Approximately 5 ml is required.
  ▪ Samples should be collected into a plain tube.

Indwelling catheters

As for **Urethral catheterization – (a) male dog**

Potential complications

As for **Urethral catheterization – (a) male dog**

U

Urethral catheterization – (c) tomcat

Indications/Use

As for **Urethral catheterization – (a) male dog**

Contraindications

As for **Urethral catheterization – (a) male dog**

Equipment

- Catheters

Catheter type	Material	Indwelling?	Sizes (Fr)	Length (cm)
Jackson cat catheter	Flexible nylon	Yes	3, 4	11
Silicone cat catheter	Medical grade silicone	Yes	3.5	12
Slippery Sam	PTFE	Yes	3, 3.5	11, 14
MILA tomcat/small animal catheter	Polyurethane	Yes	3.5, 5	15, 25

- Sterile soft gauze swabs
- Antiseptic solution: 4% chlorhexidine gluconate or 10% povidone–iodine
- Sterile gloves
- Sterile aqueous lubricant, e.g. K-Y jelly
- Plain sample pot
- Kidney dish
- 5–10 ml syringe

If the catheter is to be made indwelling:
- Suture materials; zinc oxide tape
- Sterile intravenous fluid administration set and empty fluid bag or commercial closed urine collection system, with appropriate adapters for attachment to selected urinary catheter
- Elizabethan collar

Patient preparation and positioning

- Cats usually require *heavy* sedation.
- General anaesthesia may be required for humane reasons (e.g. patient with fractured pelvis) or where catheterization is difficult (e.g. urethral obstruction).
- The patient should be restrained in lateral recumbency, with the hindlimbs pulled slightly cranially and the upper leg held away from the prepuce.
- The area around the prepuce can be clipped, especially in long-haired breeds.
- Clean the prepuce with the antiseptic, using swabs or a syringe.

Technique

1 Remove the catheter from the outer wrapper.
2 Lubricate the tip of the catheter.

3 Extrude the penis by applying gentle pressure each side of the prepuce with two fingers.

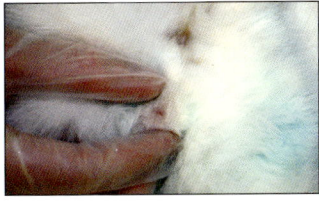
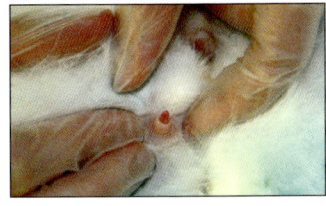

4 Gently introduce the catheter into the urethra.
5 To allow safe advancement of the catheter, the prepuce and penis should be grasped and pulled in a caudal direction to straighten out the penile and membranous urethra.

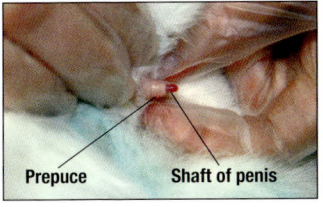

Prepuce   Shaft of penis

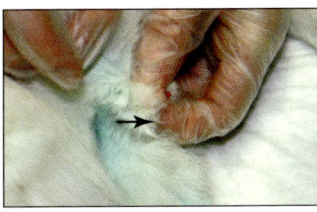

6 As soon as the catheter tip enters the bladder and urine appears in the catheter hub, advance the catheter 1 cm further. Remove stylet if present.
7 Proceed according to reason for catheterization (e.g. drain bladder, collect urine sample, administer contrast agent).

Sample handling

- For **urinalysis**:
  - Approximately 5 ml is required
  - Samples should be collected into a plain tube.

Indwelling catheters

As for **Urethral catheterization – (a) male dog**, but see Notes below.

CATHETER CHOICE

- Nylon catheters are *not* recommended for indwelling use.
- Foley catheters are *not* suitable for tomcats because of their size.
- The catheter tip should sit just within the bladder to avoid irritation of the bladder wall (too long) or urethra (too short). The MILA catheter has suture wings that can be positioned anywhere along the length of the catheter, to achieve the ideal length within the bladder.

Potential complications

As for **Urethral catheterization – (a) male dog**

Urethral catheterization – (d) tomcat with a blocked urethra

Indications/Use

- Urethral obstruction:
    - Gentle massage of the penis between the thumb and forefinger, while at the same time applying **extremely gentle** pressure to the bladder, may relieve the obstruction; if not relieved immediately, retrograde urohydropulsion should be attempted
    - Radiography may be performed to check for uroliths but, as radiolucent urethral plugs are much more common than uroliths in cats, it is not seen as a prerequisite
    - Urethral plugs or uroliths lodged in the urethra can be flushed into the bladder, to restore urethral patency

> **WARNING**
>
> - Any animal with urethral obstruction should undergo emergency assessment and stabilization, including **intravenous catheter placement**, **blood sampling – (b) venous** for an emergency minimum database, and fluid therapy for correction of acid–base and electrolyte abnormalities.
> - Bradycardia or other arrhythmias associated with hyperkalaemia should be treated aggressively.

Equipment

- A selection of urinary catheters of varying sizes (3–5 Fr) including polypropylene or silicone tomcat catheters, plastic ophthalmic lacrimal duct flush cannulas, red rubber urinary catheters, and over-the-needle intravenous catheters (23 G) without their stylet
- 3-way taps
- Intravenous extension tubing
- 10–20 ml syringes
- Antiseptic solution: 4% chlorhexidine gluconate or 10% povidone–iodine
- Sterile intravenous fluid administration set and empty fluid bag or commercial closed urine collection system, with appropriate adapters for attachment to selected urinary catheter
- Sterile isotonic fluids (e.g. saline, lactated Ringer's solution)
- Sterile water-soluble lubricant
- Elizabethan collar

Patient preparation and positioning

- General anaesthesia is most often recommended.
- Sedation should not be prolonged because of fluid, electrolyte and acid–base abnormalities.
- Positioning is as for **Urethral catheterization – (c) tomcat**.
- The prepuce is cleaned with antiseptic (excluding alcohol) and rinsed with warm water.

Technique

1   Decompress the bladder by **cystocentesis** if overdistended, using a needle attached to intravenous extension tubing, a 3-way tap and a syringe. This apparatus permits decompression without repeated puncturing of the bladder wall. The needle is held in position within the bladder, while an assistant withdraws urine. Remove as much urine as possible to avoid leakage.

2   Perform **urethral catheterization – (c) tomcat** steps 1 to 5. Flush the urethra while advancing the catheter. Gently twisting the catheter can also sometimes aid its passage. If catheterization is unsuccessful, try different/smaller types of catheter.

3   Once the catheter has been passed into the bladder, empty the bladder by attaching a syringe to the catheter.

4   Collect urine samples for **urinalysis** and culture as required. A **cystocentesis** sample is preferred for culture.

5   Slowly flush the bladder multiple times with warm sterile saline until clear, emptying the bladder each time.

Indwelling catheters

The bladder should remain catheterized if:

- Relief of the obstruction was difficult
- The urine stream is small
- The bladder was overly distended and detrusor function may be questionable
- The patient is uraemic or markedly azotaemic, and diuresis is necessary
- Post-obstructive diuresis is likely and measurement of urine output is necessary in the immediate post-obstructive phase.

1   Advance the catheter into the bladder until urine appears.

2   Then advance the catheter at least 1 cm further.

3   Secure the catheter to the patient by placing an adhesive tape butterfly around the catheter at the level of the prepuce and suturing it to the prepuce. *Alternatively,* for cat catheters with suture collars, suture the prepuce to the suture collar using the holes provided.

4   Attach a sterile intravenous administration set and empty fluid bag to the urinary catheter and maintain as a closed collection system. *Alternatively,* attach a commercial sterile closed collection urine bag to the catheter: a catheter adapter may be required. Tape the tubing of the closed collection system to the tail for additional security, to prevent accidental catheter removal.

5   For cats with feline lower urinary tract disease, the urinary catheter must usually remain in place for at least 2 days until medical management has taken effect.

6   Place an Elizabethan collar.

Potential complications

- Urethral rupture; this should be minimized by gentle technique with adequate lubrication and patience
- Inability to pass a urethral catheter into the bladder. In this situation, placement of a cystostomy tube and medical

management to decrease urethral spasm and relax the urethra should be considered. Perineal urethrostomy may be required as a salvage procedure
- Urinary tract infection
- Accidental removal of an indwelling urinary catheter
- Accidental disruption of an indwelling urinary catheter, leaving the catheter tip within the bladder

Urethral catheterization – (e) queen

Indications/Use

As for **Urethral catheterization – (a) male dog**

Contraindications

As for **Urethral catheterization – (a) male dog**

Equipment

- Catheters

Catheter type	Material	Indwelling?	Sizes (Fr)	Length (cm)
Jackson cat catheter	Flexible nylon	Yes	3, 4	11
Silicone Foley	Flexible medical-grade silicone	Yes	5	30
MILA tomcat/small animal catheter	Polyurethane	Yes	3.5, 5	15, 25

- Sterile soft gauze swabs
- Antiseptic solution: 4% chlorhexidine gluconate or 10% povidone–iodine
- Sterile gloves
- Sterile aqueous lubricant, e.g. K-Y jelly
- Otoscope (may be required)
- Plain sample pot
- Kidney dish
- 5–10 ml syringe

If the catheter is to be made indwelling:
- Suture materials; zinc oxide tape
- Sterile intravenous fluid administration set and empty fluid bag or commercial closed urine collection system, with appropriate adapters for attachment to selected urinary catheter
- Elizabethan collar

Patient preparation and positioning

- Cats usually require *heavy* sedation.
- General anaesthesia may be required for humane reasons, e.g. patient with fractured pelvis.
- The cat should be positioned in lateral recumbency (right lateral recumbency for a right-handed operator; left lateral recumbency

for a left-handed operator).

- Clean the vulva with the antiseptic to remove any discharge and surface dirt.

Technique

1 Remove the catheter from the outer wrapper and cut a feeding sleeve from the inner sterile packaging if present, to allow easy feeding of the catheter into the urethra using a 'no touch' technique. Alternatively, handle the catheter with sterile gloves.

2 Lubricate the tip of the catheter.

3 Grasp the vulval lips with your non-dominant hand, allowing your dominant hand to pass the catheter along the vestibular floor in the midline.

4 Angle the catheter ventrally, placing gentle pressure until it slips into the urethra.

PRACTICAL TIPS

- The anatomy of the queen is such that the external urethral orifice is found as a depression on the vaginal floor. This allows 'blind' urethral catheterization.
- If 'blind' catheterization fails, an otoscope may be used as a vaginoscope to identify the external urethral orifice.

5 As soon as the catheter tip enters the bladder and urine appears in the catheter hub, advance the catheter 1 cm further.

6 If using a silicone Foley, inflate the balloon once the tip of the catheter is in the bladder.

7 Proceed according to reason for catheterization (e.g. drain bladder, collect urine sample, administer contrast agent).

Sample handling

- For **urinalysis**:
  - Approximately 5 ml is required
  - Samples should be collected into a plain tube.

Indwelling catheters

As for **Urethral catheterization – (a) male dog**, but see Notes below.

CATHETER CHOICE

- Nylon catheters are *not* recommended for indwelling use.
- The catheter tip should sit just within the bladder to avoid irritation of the bladder wall (too long) or urethra (too short). The MILA catheter has suture wings which can be positioned anywhere along the length of the catheter, to achieve the ideal length within the bladder.
- Jackson cat catheters will cause irritation in the female cat, due to their length and rigidity.

Potential complications

As for **Urethral catheterization – (a) male dog**

Urethral retrograde urohydropulsion in a male dog

Indications/Use

- To flush uroliths lodged in the urethra into the bladder, to restore urethral patency
- Urethral obstruction with uroliths should be confirmed with radiography *prior* to performing retrograde urohydropulsion (see **Retrograde urethrography/vaginourethrography**)

WARNING

- **Any animal with urethral obstruction should undergo emergency assessment and stabilization, including intravenous catheter placement, blood sampling – (b) venous for an emergency minimum database, and fluid therapy for correction of acid–base and electrolyte abnormalities.**
- **Bradycardia or other arrhythmias associated with hyperkalaemia should be treated aggressively**

Equipment

- As required for **Urethral catheterization – (a) male dog**; flexible nylon urinary catheters are preferred to Foley catheters for urohydropulsion
- Hypodermic needles: 21 G, 1.5 inch
- 3-way taps
- Intravenous extension tubing
- 20–50 ml syringes
- Sterile intravenous fluid administration set and empty fluid bag or commercial closed urine collection system
- Sterile isotonic fluids (e.g. saline, lactated Ringer's solution)
- Sterile water-soluble lubricant

Patient preparation and positioning

- As required for **Urethral catheterization – (a) male dog**.
- Sedation or general anaesthesia is recommended for a patient that is alert or in pain, but may not be required for the severely depressed.
- Lateral recumbency is recommended.
- The prepuce should be cleaned and flushed with antiseptic (excluding alcohol).

Technique

1 Decompress the bladder by **cystocentesis** if overdistended, using a needle attached to intravenous extension tubing, a 3-way tap and a syringe. This apparatus permits decompression without repeated puncturing of the bladder wall. The needle is held in position within the bladder, while an assistant withdraws urine.

2 Fill one 10 ml (or 12 ml) syringe with 5 ml saline and another with 5 ml of lubricant. Attach the syringes to a 3-way tap and use this to mix them.

3 Insert a lubricated large-bore male dog urinary catheter into the urethra (see **Urethral catheterization – (a) male dog**).

4 Instil 3–8 ml of the lubricant mixture around the uroliths. The tip of the catheter should remain distal to the uroliths. **Never attempt to force uroliths retrograde with the tip of the catheter.**

5 An assistant inserts a gloved index finger into the rectum and occludes the urethral lumen by compressing the urethra against the floor of the bony pelvis.

6 With a moistened gauze swab, occlude the distal urethra by compressing the distal tip of the penis around the urinary catheter.

7 Fill a large syringe (20 or 50 ml) with sterile isotonic solution. As a guide, the normal bladder will accommodate approximately 7–11 ml/kg bodyweight, but this volume is most often not required.

8 Attach the syringe to the urinary catheter.

9 Push sterile isotonic solution into the urethra, with the goal of dilating the urethral lumen around the uroliths.

10 Once the urethra is dilated, immediately release digital compression of the pelvic urethra.

11 Continue flushing fluid through the urinary catheter and urethral lumen to propel uroliths into the urinary bladder. Repeated occlusion of the pelvic urethra and flushing of the urethra may be required. Use caution not to overdistend the bladder lumen with fluid. Palpate the bladder regularly to check for overdistension and repeat bladder decompression if required.

12 Confirm successful retrograde urohydropulsion of uroliths into the bladder by **retrograde urethrography**.

13 If the animal is not taken to surgery immediately for removal of uroliths from the bladder, placement of an indwelling urethral catheter is recommended pending surgery, to maintain urine flow.

Potential complications

- Urethral rupture (rare)
- Urinary tract infection

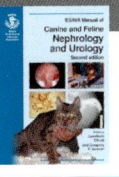

FURTHER INFORMATION

Further information on urolithiasis and its treatment can be found in the *BSAVA Manual of Canine and Feline Nephrology and Urology*.

Urinalysis

Indications/Use

- To obtain information from urine samples

> ### SAMPLE CHOICES
>
> - Cystocentesis samples are best used for culture; if this is not possible a catheter sample can be used for culture if collected aseptically but this carries a risk of contamination.
> - Cystocentesis or catheter samples are suitable for sediment analysis, urine specific gravity (SG) determination and dipstick analysis.
> - Free-catch samples are generally suitable for dipstick and SG, and are of limited use for sediment examination. They are not suitable for culture.

Equipment

- Urine sample in a plain container, obtained by **cystocentesis** or **urethral catheterization** or by free catch
- Urine sample in a *sterile* plain container collected by **cystocentesis**
- Refractometer
- Dipsticks and results chart
- Distilled water
- Syringe
- Centrifuge
- Plastic disposable pipette
- Microscope slides and coverslips
- Gloves
- Microscope

Specific gravity

Urine SG should be measured using a refractometer. Urine SG can be determined by some dipsticks but this is very unreliable and not recommended.

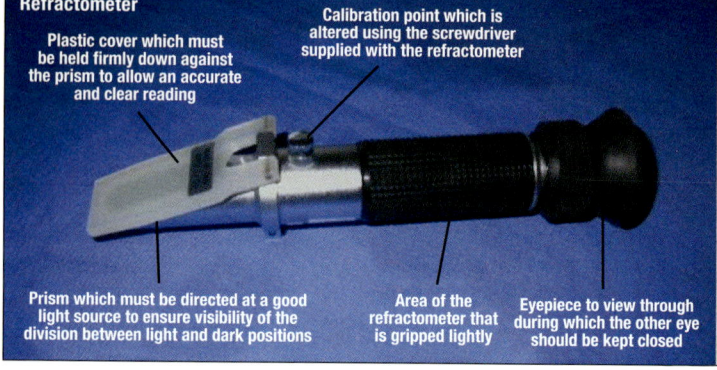

Refractometer

Plastic cover which must be held firmly down against the prism to allow an accurate and clear reading

Calibration point which is altered using the screwdriver supplied with the refractometer

Prism which must be directed at a good light source to ensure visibility of the division between light and dark positions

Area of the refractometer that is gripped lightly

Eyepiece to view through during which the other eye should be kept closed

Technique

1 Open the prism cover.
2 Check calibration of the refractometer using distilled water. This should read 1.000; if it does not, recalibrate as follows:
   i Unscrew the fixation nut of the calibration screw.
   ii Turn the calibration screw downwards to bring the scale up, or unscrew to bring the scale down until it reads 1.000.
   iii Re-affix the calibration nut.

3 To view, hold the refractometer horizontally in the direction of a good light source, preferably a natural light source.

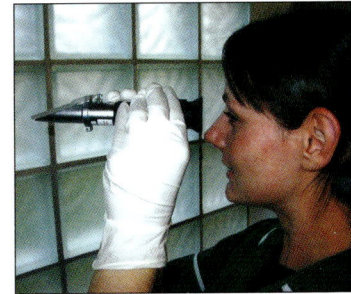

4 Wearing gloves, place 1–2 drops of urine on the face of the lower prism and view through the eyepiece. Note where the colour boundary line is and read against the specific gravity scale.

5 After use, clean the prism and cover carefully with a soft wet cloth or damp lens wipe.

Dipstick tests

These constitute a qualitative to semiquantitative method of monitoring major chemicals of interest in the urine. The dipsticks are designed for monitoring constituents in human urine; therefore, some of the tests are not suitable for use with animal urine, i.e. SG, nitrite and leucocyte esterase activity (WBC).

Technique

- Only fresh, in-date sticks should be used. Dipsticks should be stored in the original tightly capped container (the lid contains dessicant).
- Fresh urine should be used.

1 Do not touch the test pads with fingers.
2 Dip the urine test strip in fresh urine and tap off any excess.
   Alternatively, use a syringe to place drops of urine on each test pad. Allow excess urine to run off.

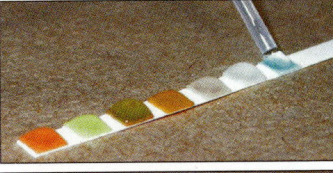

3 Check the colour changes at the indicated times.
4 Compare the strip with the test chart provided.

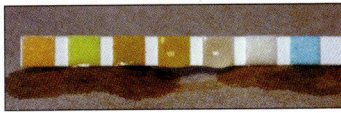

Urine sediment analysis

This is perhaps the most important component of a complete routine urinalysis. A suggested method for preparation and analysis is as follows:

1 Use fresh urine or refrigerated urine that has been warmed to room temperature. Note that storage periods of longer than a few hours may have detrimental effects on cellular elements.

2 Mix the sample well but gently, to prevent destruction of any casts.

3 Place a constant volume (10, 5 or 3 ml; often 3 ml is used for cat urine), in a conical centrifuge tube.

4 Gently centrifuge the urine (approximately 1000 rpm for 5 minutes, though this will vary with the type of centrifuge used). If a smaller volume of urine (i.e. <3 ml) is used with high speed centrifugation, the amount of sediment obtained may be too small, especially if the urine is very dilute. The high speed may also damage cells and destroy casts.

5 Decant most of the supernatant (this can be used in the refractometer for SG analysis – see above).

6 A few drops of liquid will remain in the tube. Sediment is mixed in this to resuspend it, either by gently tapping the tube or pipetting up and down.

7 If a specialized urine stain, such as Sedistain, is being used, add 1 drop to the sediment and mix.

8 Place a drop of sediment on a clean microscope slide and place a coverslip over it, avoiding air bubbles.

9 Place the slide on the microscope stage and scan the whole area on low power (10X objective). If unstained sediment is being used, lower the condenser until there is good resolution.

10 Report the presence of crystals at this magnification.

11 Change the objective to high power (40X) and rescan the area. Count and record the numbers of erythrocytes, leucocytes, epithelial cells, casts, crystals and bacteria seen per high power field. It is advisable to count in 5–10 different fields and then calculate an average unless there are very large numbers seen.

12 Report other constituents, e.g. spermatozoa, mucus strands, yeast, fungi, nematode eggs, fat droplets.

13 For further identification of cell types or to differentiate bacteria from particles, use the 100X oil immersion objective. Distinguish fat and air bubbles by fine focusing and moving the condenser. Distinguish Brownian motion of particles from motile bacteria at 100X power.

Bacterial culture

Cystocentesis samples are best for culture. Samples collected by free catch or catheterization are contaminated by the resident bacterial flora from the mid-urethra to the external genitalia. In dogs, bacterial contamination occurs in up to 85% of voided midstream samples and up to 26% of catheterized samples; contamination is greater in samples from bitches than in those from male dogs.

1   Collect approximately 5 ml of urine in a sterile plain tube. **Note that the use of a container containing boric acid preservative (red top universal container) is no longer recommended if samples are to be transported to a laboratory for analysis.**

2   Analyse as soon as possible after collection. If the sample has to be transported to an external laboratory, ideally it should be analysed within 24 hours of collection.

FURTHER INFORMATION

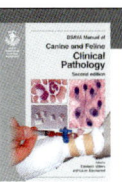

Information on interpretation of urinalysis, and illustrations of sediment inclusions, can be found in the *BSAVA Manual of Canine and Feline Clinical Pathology*.

U

Velpeau sling

Indications/Use

- To hold the shoulder, elbow and carpus in flexion, supporting the forelimb in a non-weight-bearing position
- Immobilizes the shoulder to promote healing of shoulder and scapula injuries, including traumatic medial shoulder luxation and minimally displaced scapular fractures

Equipment

- Padded bandage material or cast padding
- Conforming gauze bandage
- Outer protective bandaging material, e.g. self-adhesive non-adherent bandage

Patient preparation and positioning

- Manual support, with the animal in a standing position on three legs, is often all that is required.
- Sedation or general anaesthesia may be required for a non-compliant animal.

Technique

1 Lightly pad the antebrachium with a padded bandage material.

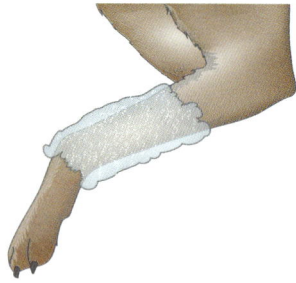

2 Secure the padded bandage material to the antebrachium with conforming gauze bandage, working in a medial to dorsal to lateral direction.

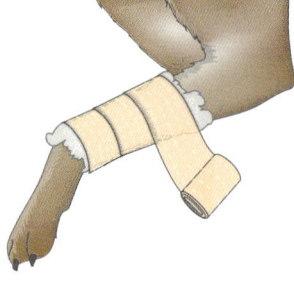

3 Gently flex the elbow and shoulder. Pass the conforming gauze bandage from the medial aspect of the antebrachium, across the lateral aspects of the humerus and scapula, to the dorsal aspect of the thorax.

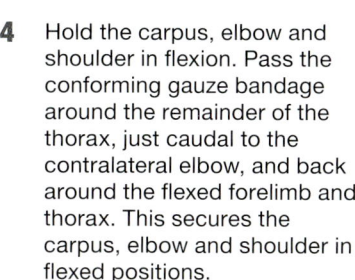

4 Hold the carpus, elbow and shoulder in flexion. Pass the conforming gauze bandage around the remainder of the thorax, just caudal to the contralateral elbow, and back around the flexed forelimb and thorax. This secures the carpus, elbow and shoulder in flexed positions.

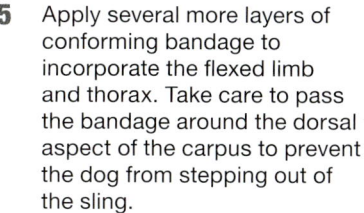

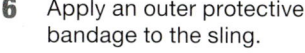

5 Apply several more layers of conforming bandage to incorporate the flexed limb and thorax. Take care to pass the bandage around the dorsal aspect of the carpus to prevent the dog from stepping out of the sling.

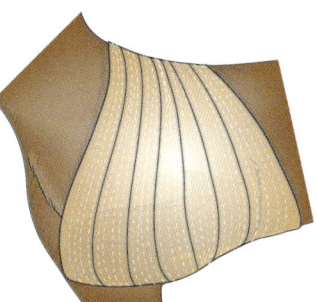

6 Apply an outer protective bandage to the sling.

NOTES

- The technique above has been described as a 'non-weight-bearing' sling and may be appropriate for traumatic lateral shoulder luxations. However, velpeau slings may promote reluxation of unstable traumatic lateral shoulder luxations.
- In the case of medial shoulder luxations, adduction of the humerus against the thoracic wall is most important to give external rotation of the shoulder. Therefore, it may be preferable to bandage the humerus against the thoracic wall prior to incorporating the rest of the flexed limb in the bandage.

A
B
C
D
E
F
G
H
I
J
K
L
M
N
O
P
Q
R
S
T
U
V
W
X
Y
Z

Sling maintenance

- The sling is maintained for 2–6 weeks for traumatic shoulder luxations managed conservatively.
- Velpeau slings should be checked every 4 hours for the first 24 hours, and at least twice daily thereafter for complications.

Potential complications

- If applied too tightly, potential complications include:
    - Limb swelling due to venous stasis
    - Irritation of the skin, especially of the contralateral axillary region
    - Pressure necrosis of the soft tissues
    - Excessive flexion of the carpus, resulting in discomfort and/or trauma to the antebrachium from the claws
    - Respiratory compromise
- If the sling becomes wet, moist dermatitis and soft tissue maceration may occur
- Velpeau sling loosening results in the animal stepping out of the sling

Water deprivation test

Indications/Use

Diagnostic aid in cases of:

- Central diabetes insipidus
- Primary nephrogenic diabetes insipidus
- Primary (psychogenic) polydipsia

Contraindications

- Dehydration
- Azotaemia
- Pyometra
- Pyelonephritis
- Hypercalcaemia
- Hyperadrenocorticism

> **WARNING**
>
> - The water deprivation test should be performed only after all other causes of polyuria and polydipsia have been ruled out, limiting the differential diagnoses to central diabetes insipidus, primary nephrogenic diabetes insipidus and psychogenic polydipsia.
> - Failure to recognize the more common polyuric syndromes such as pyometra, pyelonephritis, early renal insufficiency, hypercalcaemia or hyperadrenocorticism may lead to an incorrect or inconclusive diagnosis and *use of the water deprivation test in these patients may be dangerous.*

Equipment

- Urinary catheter
- Electronic scales
- Measuring vessel for water
- Refractometer
- Intravenous desmopressin (DDAVP) (synthetic analogue of antidiuretic hormone (ADH))
- 2 ml syringes
- Hypodermic needles: 21 G, ¾ to 1 inch

Technique

It is recommended that the water deprivation test be performed in three consecutive stages:

1. Gradual water restriction.
2. Followed immediately by abrupt water deprivation.
3. Followed immediately by an antidiuretic hormone (ADH) response test – if necessary.

Stage 1 – Gradual water restriction

To minimize the effects of renal medullary washout on test results, progressive water restriction is recommended *before* abrupt water deprivation. This is usually carried out by the owner in the home environment.

The *owner* should:

1 Begin reducing the amount of water provided to the animal 3 days before the abrupt water deprivation test is to be performed in the clinic.
2 During the first 24 hours, allow the dog or cat twice its normal daily water requirement (120–150 ml/kg) divided into 6–8 small portions.
3 During the next 24 hours, give 80–100 ml/kg.
4 Over the last 24 hours, give 60–80 ml/kg.
5 During the 3-day period of gradual water restriction, owners should feed dry food and monitor the animal's bodyweight on a daily basis.
6 Owners should also be instructed to observe for any significant decrease in the animal's mentation when performing gradual water deprivation. **Should this occur the test should be stopped and veterinary attention sought immediately**.

Stage 2 – Abrupt water deprivation

The goal of stage 2 is to achieve maximal ADH secretion and concentration of urine. This would be expected to occur after a 3–5% loss of bodyweight. **This procedure must be carried out in the veterinary clinic** and is best started early in the day.

1 Completely empty the animal's bladder (see **Urethral catheterization**; consider an indwelling urinary catheter, especially in females) and collect the urine.
2 Record the urine specific gravity (SG; see **Urinalysis**), obtain an exact bodyweight and remove all food and water.
3 At 1–2 hourly intervals, again completely empty the animal's bladder, measure the urine SG and reweigh the animal (to monitor for dehydration).
4 Continue until there is *either* a 5% loss in bodyweight *or* the urine SG is >1.030 in dogs or >1.035 in cats. The major difficulty with the water deprivation test is that its duration can never be predicted accurately.

> **WARNING**
> - **The animal must also be monitored for signs of CNS depression. *Stop the test immediately if these are seen.***

5 Some animals will fail to reach the 5% dehydration endpoint by the end of the working day. In this situation, the patient can be transferred to a facility with overnight care so that monitoring of urine SG and bodyweight can continue overnight.

Alternatively, overnight access to water in maintenance amounts (2.5–3.0 ml/kg/h) can be provided; the following morning, water is once again withdrawn and monitoring continued until a 5% loss of bodyweight or the target urine SG is reached.

Stage 3 – Response to intravenous desmopressin

If the dog or cat has lost 5% or more of its original bodyweight after water deprivation, but the urine SG remains <1.015, an ADH (desmopressin) response test should be performed in the clinic, again early in the day if possible.

1 Provide water in maintenance amounts (2.5–3.0 ml/kg/h) for the duration of this stage.
2 Intravenously inject desmopressin (DDAVP):
   - 2.0 μg (**micrograms**) for dogs <15 kg and cats
   - 4.0 μg (**micrograms**) for dogs >15 kg.
3 Completely empty the animal's bladder (see **Urethral catheterization**; consider an indwelling urinary catheter, especially in females) and collect the urine.
4 Record the urine SG (see **Urinalysis**) every 1 hour.
5 Stop the test when the urine SG has risen above 1.015 or the animal shows any signs of CNS depression.
6 Continue this stage for a maximum of 10 hours.
7 Upon completion of the test, water should be offered in maintenance amounts (2.5–3.0 ml/kg/h) for 2–3 hours then provided *ad libitum*.

Results

Disorder	Urine SG prior to test	Urine SG after stage 2	Urine SG after stage 3
Central diabetes insipidus (complete)	1.001–1.007	<1.008	Increase to >1.010–1.015
Central diabetes insipidus (partial)	1.001–1.007	1.008–1.020	Increase to >1.015
Primary nephrogenic diabetes insipidus	1.001–1.007	<1.008	No change (remains <1.008)
Primary polydipsia	1.001–1.020	>1.030	No additional increase

Potential complications

- Severe dehydration has the potential to lead to renal failure
- Rapid rehydration following the end of the test has the potential to result in cerebral oedema and neurological signs

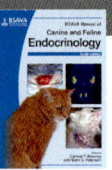
Whole blood clotting time

Indications/Use

- Assessment of secondary haemostasis (intrinsic and common pathways). Note that the whole blood clotting time (WBCT) will also be prolonged in severe thrombocytopenia and hypofibrinogenaemia.

NOTES

- WBCT is a relatively insensitive test of secondary haemostasis, and is only prolonged when a factor is depleted to <5% of its normal level. It is also influenced by other variables, such as the volume of blood, haematocrit, tube size, temperature and tube coating (plastic *versus* glass). Due to these considerations this test is not recommended for routine use.
- In an emergency situation, a prolonged WBCT suggests a severe coagulopathy; for example, due to anticoagulant rodenticide toxicosis, particularly in those animals with a high clinical index of suspicion for this disorder.
- If the WBCT is within the reference interval, a haemostatic disorder may still be present, and more specific coagulation tests such as prothrombin time or partial thromboplastin time should be assessed.

Equipment

- Hypodermic needles:
  - Cats: 21–23 G; $^5/_8$ inch
  - Dogs: 21 G; $^5/_8$ or 1 inch
- 2 ml and 5 ml syringes
- 70% surgical spirit
- 4% chlorhexidine gluconate or 10% povidone–iodine
- Cotton wool or gauze swabs
- 10 ml plain glass tube (no anticoagulant)
- Stopwatch or timer

Technique

1 Blood is collected from the *jugular vein* (see **Blood sampling – (b) venous**).

- To minimize contamination with tissue factor, collect the first 0.5 ml of blood into a syringe and discard, but keep the needle in the vein.
- Draw approximately 4.5 ml of blood into a new syringe.

2 Place the blood into the tube and start a stopwatch or timer.

3 Keep the tube warm by holding it in the palm of the hand.

4 Tip gently to 90 degrees every 30 seconds until the blood has coagulated.

5 Stop the stopwatch/timer and note the time taken for the blood to clot.

Reference ranges

Reported reference intervals are:

- Dogs: <13 minutes
- Cats: <8 minutes

List of abbreviations

ACD	Acid citrate dextrose
ACTH	Adrenocorticotropic hormone
ALS	Advanced life support
APTT	Activated partial thromboplastin time
BAL	Bronchoalveolar lavage
BLS	Basic life support
BMBT	Buccal mucosal bleeding time
CCL	Cranial cruciate ligament
CNS	Central nervous system
CPA	Cardiopulmonary arrest
CPD	Citrate phosphate dextrose
CPDA	Citrate phosphate dextrose adenine
CPR	Cardiopulmonary resuscitation
CSF	Cerebrospinal fluid
CT	Computed tomography
DPL	Diagnostic peritoneal lavage
DV	Dorsoventral
ECG	Electrocardiography
EDTA	Ethylene diamine tetra-acetic acid
ET	Endotracheal
ETCO$_2$	End-tidal carbon dioxide
GI	Gastrointestinal
HAC	Hyperadrenocorticism
LMN	Lower motor neuron
MRI	Magnetic resonance imaging
OSPT	One-stage prothrombin time
P_aCO_2	Partial pressure of carbon dioxide in arterial blood
P_aO_2	Partial pressure of oxygen in arterial blood
PCV	Packed cell volume
PD	Peritoneal dialysis
RER	Resting energy requirement
S_pO_2	Oxygen saturation in peripheral capillary blood
TP	Total protein
UMN	Upper motor neuron
VD	Ventrodorsal
WBCT	Whole blood clotting time

Index

Page numbers in *italic* type indicate illustrations.

INDEX